An Introduction to Herbalism

*Step into Nature's Healing—From Growing
Your Own Medicine to Crafting Herbal Teas
for Vibrant Well-being*

The Green Glow

Contents

Freebies For Our Supporters!

We've got a nice beginner recipe book for all of you herbal newbies out there. Just scan the code below to claim yours!

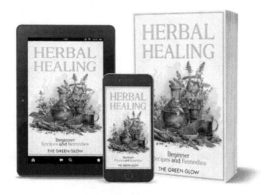

I want my freebie!

Join Our Budding Community!

We have a brand new community and we want **YOU** to help us grow! Are you willing to be one of the first seeds in our Facebook garden? Do you have any questions? Do you want share your herbal world with us and our glowing community? If you answered yes to any of these then, well, what are you waiting for? Just scan the code to join our community!

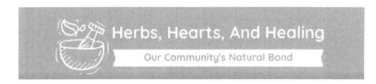

Introduction
The World of Herbalism

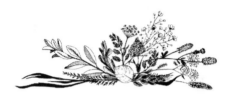

The greatest medicine of all is teaching people how not to need it.

— Hippocrates

Welcome, dear reader! Here, we start our engaging exploration into the fascinating world of herbalism. Are you ready? It's quite the journey. Who is this book for? You might be a seasoned herbalist looking to refresh your knowledge, a complete beginner keen to learn more, or someone looking to understand better what natural health is. Everyone is welcome here!

Today, herbal medicine is one of the most well-known examples of holistic health and natural remedies, combining age-old wisdom with innovative technology breakthroughs. The ancient practice is centered on using plant extracts for therapeutic purposes and transcends many cultures over time, reflecting our never-ending search for natural health remedies! To better understand herbalism, we need to look at the past, where it all started, how it can be used, and the complex relationship it shares with our more modern medical perspectives.

It's rather incredible how this ancient practice still remains so relevant today. But if we think about how our fast-paced modern world is scattered with synthetic medicines and other quick fixes, it's no wonder why so many individuals are opting to return to greener roots. We want a healthier way of caring for ourselves while keeping it as natural as possible, right? Plants possess the just healing powers we need!

So, with herbalism dating back to the start of human civilization, we glimpse its importance by looking at the ancient Egyptians, the Chinese, the indigenous people of America, and even European apothecaries during the Middle Ages... The list is endless, but luckily, we have a whole chapter dedicated to exploring the landscapes and cultures herbalism, also often referred to as traditional medicine, has touched. The wisdom has been passed down from generation to generation, including specific treatments and a way of looking at our health and well-being in general. The World Health Organization (WHO) explains traditional medicine is all the knowledge, skills, and practices that are based on native theories, beliefs, and experiences and are used in many cultures to keep individuals healthy and to prevent, diagnose, improve, or even treat various physical and mental illnesses (World Health Organization, 2019).

Something delicate lies between the respectful ways of doing things from the past and the harsh realities of modern pharmaceutical therapies. This bridge is made of more than just time. It's also made of knowing and switching between how we view things. Our reliance on what is immediate, practical, and (often) synthetic has increased as our civilizations have progressed. We swapped hours of drying herbs in the sun for one minute at the drugstore checkout. But as we dig deeper, we start to see a theme that arises: a desire for authenticity. The story, which is as old as society itself, is not meant to downplay the progress made in modern medicine. Instead, it is intended to show how these discoveries can be used alongside ancient wisdom, where modern science and old herbal practices meet. Guess what? We have arrived! We are on the verge of rediscovering and redefining what health is.

As our story continues, we notice a significant change in how people think about their well-being these days. We soon realized that our modern medicines have some limitations alongside unwanted side effects. Think nausea, dizzy spells, and dry mouths (which is the least of our problems on that list).

It's become too easy to purchase that packet of pain pills and drink a few when we experience discomfort. It's like we revert to auto-pilot whenever we feel uncomfortable. Quick! What is the fastest way to feel at ease again? Think about it: We have a minor (or major) headache. What do we do? We immediately seek relief and reach for that medication. Did you ever stop to think whether there was a more natural way of getting rid of the pain? Because there is. The recent revival of herbalism can be linked to the increasing popularity of organic and natural lifestyles and a growing emphasis on wellness and one's own well-being. This comeback is not a passing trend but a more intentional shift toward person-centered, environmentally conscious, and body-honoring health solutions.

While herbalism has a long history, it has grown increasingly integrated with modern medicine in the twenty-first century. According to the National Centre for Complementary and Integrative Health (NCCIH), herbal supplements are critical to modern herbal medicine. These supplements complement one's diet and contain therapeutically useful herbs or botanicals (National Centre for Complementary and Integrative Health, 2023).

Herbalism has many applications but still has complicated legal and safety issues. For example, the Food and Drug Administration (FDA) in the United States establishes specific dietary supplement guidelines. These guidelines help us to draw attention to the regulatory and supervisory differences between prescription or over-the-counter drugs and nutritional supplements. Therefore, given that herbal medicines currently on the market cannot pass the stringent testing and standardization requirements for pharmaceuticals, herbalists and consumers (this is us) are urged to use our discretion and always be well-informed about the herbal products we purchase (National Centre for Complementary and Integrative Health, 2023). Something worth noting: It's always safer to consult your medical practitioner before making any changes to your diet or lifestyle, as we all respond differently to specific remedies. This includes the advice and guidance offered in this book.

It can be exciting to try something new, but we need to be cautious of the quantity and, most notably, the quality of our products. These dynamics make it more evident how relevant, trustworthy, and empirically based information is. Groups like the American Botanical Council (ABC) are leading this effort, which shares invaluable specifics on herbs and medicinal plants that have undergone in-depth analysis and evaluation by subject-matter experts. Their knowledge-sharing endeavors are intended to close the gap between conventional wisdom and modern science so that herbal treatments have a reliable foundation (American Botanical Council, 2023).

The ABC represents a more significant trend toward evidence-based herbalism, together with other groups of a similar kind. By integrating historical customs with cutting-edge scientific research, they aim to legitimize and enhance the use of herbs in medicine. This approach takes herbalism from mythology and stories to verified health research, which helps demystify the practice (especially for individuals starting). These organizations educate the public and medical professionals by emphasizing safety, effectiveness, and responsible use and support the idea that herbal medicines should become more widely accepted and integrated into traditional medical practice.

However, herbalism is much more than drinking tablets or liquids. It is a living, dynamic art that calls for a close relationship with the plant world and an innate understanding of the medicinal value that plants offer. Like in other contexts, such as kitchens, gardens, and natural settings, where people cultivate, harvest, and prepare plants in various ways, they engage with plants directly. Like the plants, the uses are diverse, from essential oils and beverages designed from therapeutic herbs to romantic and soothing herbal baths (and occasionally to spice up our latest dinner recipes). In addition to encouraging a greater degree of respect and a deeper connection with nature, this interactive aspect of herbalism educates us to take charge of our health, both inside and out.

Furthermore, the process of creating herbal medicines is person-centered. Herbal medicines can be customized to match your unique needs by considering factors such as your body, lifestyle, and pre-existing medical concerns, as opposed to the one-size-fits-all approach we see in conventional medicine. This individualization reflects a core principle of herbalism, which views healing and health as a personalized, holistic journey rather than just treating symptoms. You get to grow your medicine in the comfort of your home!

With all that said, herbalism has a bright future ahead of it, filled with possibilities and challenges as the twenty-first century progresses. Due to advancements in technology, more scientific support, and a growing focus on sustainable healthcare, herbal medicine will indeed become increasingly important in the future of world health. A well-balanced and thoughtful strategy for growing this practice is necessary since, at the same time, problems like quality control, ecological sustainability of plant resources, and the need for more widespread education and regulation continue.

Intending to enlighten, educate, and inspire you, this book embarks on an exciting journey throughout this extensive topic. These pages offer a thorough summary, practical tips, and a greater understanding of herbalism. This book will guide you on using herbs beyond fancy infused teas (we'll do that, too!). It's here to teach you precisely what herbalism is, how it has taken shape in the last few years (if not centuries), how you can successfully grow your own herb garden, and all the fascinating ways you can integrate herbs into your daily life. In our final chapter, we'll also explore how you can find your community of herbalists! Together, we'll appreciate the wisdom in herbs and plants as we flip each page and learn how to use their healing powers sustainably and ethically for our (and the planet's) well-being.

Chapter 1

The Rich Tapestry of Herbal History

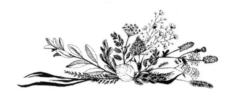

The art of healing comes from nature, not from the physician. Therefore the physician must start from nature, with an open mind.

— Paracelsus

Welcome to the unfolding narrative of herbal medicine. This journey is more than just an exploration of plants and their uses; it's an odyssey that spans millennia, encompassing cultural revolutions, deep-rooted wisdom, and, sometimes, radical shifts from conventional practices. The adventure we're on here isn't simply an intellectual stroll but a dynamic, informative adventure into how plants have shaped health and healing throughout different cultures.

The Origins of Herbal Medicine

Ancient Egyptian civilization, renowned for its tremendous architecture and complex hieroglyphs, was also extraordinarily progressive in its medical practices. Egyptian medicine uncovers a rich legacy that welcomed not only advanced surgical procedures and public health systems but also a philosophy that interconnected physical health with spiritual beliefs and the afterlife. Such a nuanced understanding of herbal remedies, blended seamlessly into everyday life, presents us with invaluable insights into the early chapters of herbal medicine.

The Ebers Papyrus and Beyond

Some 5,000 years ago, the bustling banks of the Nile were the cradle of not just architectural wonders but also of medical breakthroughs. The Ebers Papyrus, dating back to around 1500 B.C.E., is a pivotal witness to this era. It is one of the first complete medical records and contains just over 700 herbal prescriptions and treatments, revealing the Egyptians' extensive knowledge and use of medicinal plants. Ingredients such as aloe, garlic, juniper, and basil were used to address a spectrum of conditions, ranging from common digestive disorders to more complicated illnesses (Moorhouse, 2018; Pan et al., 2014; *The History of Herbal Medicine*, 2020). These are some of the very herbs we have in our kitchens today! Does anyone need a basil-infused remedy for an ancient touch of wellness?

Integration of Medicine and Religion

Have you ever thought about how our ancestors approached healing? It wasn't just about the physical symptoms. Take the ancient Egyptians, for instance. They didn't see medicine as we do today. For them, it was intertwined with their spiritual and religious beliefs. Textual evidence from both the Ebers Papyrus and the Edwin Smith Papyrus catalogs the variety of medicines and concoctions used but also outlines the accompanying chants and prayers. The merging of the physical and spiritual domains highlights an all-encompassing approach to treatment, where well-being is defined as a balance of body, mind, and spiritual harmony. How different would our modern healthcare be if we were treated with such a holistic approach?

Surgical Expertise and Public Health

Aside from their knowledge of herbal mixtures, the ancient Egyptians pioneered surgical treatments and public health advancements. They certainly exceeded our expectations. Surgical treatises like the Edwin Smith Papyrus reveal astonishingly advanced techniques, some of which remain impressive even by our modern standards. Moorhouse (2018) observes that the Egyptians' medical and surgical expertise was complemented by pioneering public health measures, including systems for water sanitation and waste disposal, evidencing a foresight in public health and hygiene far ahead of its era. Would ancient Egyptian surgeons be amazed or amused by our contemporary operating rooms?

Comparative Perspective and Legacy

Comparing the medical methodologies of the Egyptians with those of the next civilizations, like the Roman Empire, reveals both continuities and variations within the medical field. Egyptian medical thought was compelling, especially when it came to herbal medicine. They had foundational principles that later cultures embraced, modified, and advanced. It's incredible how their ideas influenced others. They valued their herbal practice, which went beyond traditional treatments. It was a system that brought together physical health, spiritual understanding, and community. Their sophisticated use of medicinal plants, combined with their advancements in surgical techniques and a well-organized public health structure, demonstrate a holistic view of medicine that is as captivating as it is instructional.

Neanderthals to Hippocrates: The Herbal Continuum

Did you know that our ancestors, even the Neanderthals, have been using medicinal plants for a long time? It's fascinating how profoundly rooted this practice is in our history. Archaeologists have discovered interesting evidence about Neanderthals, which includes remnants of yarrow, chamomile, and poplar at Neanderthal sites, suggesting that these early humans used different plants for medicinal reasons. It's fascinating to think about how people from over 60,000 years ago already had a natural understanding of how certain plants could heal. They knew that certain herbs had anti-inflammatory and pain-relieving properties. This discovery highlights the practical use of plants for health but also an early cognitive connection to nature and an early awareness of its potential to aid in healing and maintaining well-being (*The History of Herbal Medicine*, 2020).

The vast growth of herbal knowledge is signified in ancient Greece by the legendary physician Hippocrates, often called the "Father of Medicine." Hippocrates truly was ahead of his time! He believed in the power of observing natural causes and treatments for diseases, which was a significant change from the superstitious and mystical explanations that were widespread back then. He also had the innate knowledge that herbs can heal. One of his favorites was Willow bark, a remarkable salicylic acid compound, which is similar to the main ingredient in aspirin that we use today. His philosophy on healthcare can be witnessed through one of his very own sayings, "Let food be thy medicine, and medicine be thy food." This illustrates how important he believed our diet and natural remedies were for staying healthy. This enduring wisdom shows us how herbal medicine has been essential in healthcare for quite some time. It also shows how the medical field has changed and still affects our healthcare practices today. Some of Hippocrates' principles have laid the groundwork for a more holistic and balanced approach to health, integrating the natural healing power of herbs, and continue to resonate and inform modern herbal medicine and dietary practices (*The History of Herbal Medicine*, 2020).

Herbal Traditions Around the World

The practice of herbalism, essential to traditional medicine around the globe, uses around 350,000 different plant species. Beyond historical attraction, there is a modern return to this innate plant knowledge. It is recognized for its effectiveness, having minimal side effects, and its critical role in preventing microbial resistance to synthetic medications. This section will glimpse into some of the most significant and influential herbal traditions around the globe. Ancient texts, here we come.

Chinese Herbal Medicine

In China, the legendary emperor Shen Nong, often revered as the father of Chinese agriculture, is renowned for his monumental contributions to traditional Chinese medicine (TCM). Believed to have lived around 2500 B.C.E., Shen Nong is credited with tasting hundreds of herbs and identifying their medicinal properties, laying the foundation for using herbs in Chinese healing practices. Much later, around 250 CE, these findings and teachings were methodically gathered in the ancient text *Shennong Ben Cao Jing*. This book is considered a cornerstone of traditional Chinese medicine because it organizes and discusses many plants and their medicinal characteristics and applications. It represents an enormous leap forward in herbal documentation and has played an instrumental role in shaping the course of Chinese herbal therapy, influencing not just China but also the broader Asian region (Pan et al., 2014). Because of its large and diverse geography, China is home to 31,000 plant species, which reflects its incredible biodiversity. Both indigenous and imported herbs are used in medicine because of these abundant natural resources and rich historical background. Today, China has a considerable effect on the global herbal industry, as evidenced by the approximately 8,000 Chinese herbal treatments sold to other countries.

The Indian Ayurvedic System

While Egypt and China were developing their medical systems, the Indian subcontinent wasn't far behind with its Ayurveda, dating back to around 3300 BCE. We're free to imagine a lifestyle where herbs are not just add-ons but essential elements of daily life. Ayurveda, literally the "science of life," is all about a balanced lifestyle–good food, yoga, meditation, and, of course, herbs. Their go-to guide is the "Charaka Samhita," attributed to the wise sage Charaka. Think of it as an ancient encyclopedia detailing thousands of plants and their uses in healing. This text doesn't only list remedies; it's about syncing your body, mind, and spirit for overall wellness. And guess what? The age-old wisdom in the "Charaka Samhita" isn't outdated; it's very much alive, influencing holistic health practices globally (Pan et al., 2014). Indian medicine is led by the philosophy that "everything can be a drug." They have about 45,000 plant species and 3,500 of those are for healing.

The European Chapter: Renaissance and Rebellion

During the Renaissance, Europe's herbal history took a turn. Influential works like Banckes's Herbal (1525) and Grete Herball (1526) emerged, shifting herbal wisdom into the mainstream. These books, written in the local tongues instead of elite Latin, brought herbs such as Rosemary and Chamomile into regular households, encouraging their use for day-to-day health and common ailments (*The History of Herbal Medicine*, 2020).

Nicholas Culpeper, an English botanist and herbalist, played a definitive role during this period. He was known for questioning established medical norms and focusing on distributing medical and herbal knowledge to the masses. His essential work, *The Complete Herbal*, published in 1653, was not in Latin but in straightforward English, making the subject of herbs that much more approachable and practical to the general public. Culpeper's comprehensive insights, combined with his personal experience, make "The Complete Herbal" a timeless resource in herbal medicine, appreciated for its real-world applications and because it's easy to understand (*The History of Herbal Medicine*, 2020).

Herbalism in the New World

As the Americas opened their doors to the world through colonization, the narrative of herbalism became a rich blend of indigenous, African, and European traditions. The herbal knowledge of Native Americans, especially, turned out to be a lifeline for European settlers. These indigenous populations brought various new therapeutic approaches and medicines, setting the stage for cultural interchange.

A noteworthy mention of the women in these cultures—their contributions during this historical era are particularly influential. Whether among indigenous communities or the new settlers, it was typically women who were responsible for the identification, collection, and preparation of medical herbs. This crucial responsibility placed them at the heart of health and wellness in their communities; their intimate knowledge of plant-based healing bridged gaps between cultures and ensured the well-being of their societies, highlighting an often-over-looked aspect of healthcare in these transformative times.

Modern Twists and Turns

The winding path herbalism has taken throughout the centuries has not always been as insightful and pleasant. Take the Salem Witch Trials in the 17th century, for instance. A misinterpreta-tion and fear of herbal and natural healing practices partly fueled these infamous trials. As we flash forward to the early 20th century, we see the surprise of the pharmaceutical industry and a move toward uniform medical education. This shift placed herbalism on the back burner, often dismissing it as mere folklore rather than a legitimate medical practice (*The History of Herbal Medicine*, 2020).

But here is the plot twist: The last few decades have seen a vibrant renewal of interest in herbal medicine. This revival isn't just a whimsical throwback. It responds to the rising frustration with traditional healthcare and its potential risks. The crucial factor is that an abundance of scientific study is supporting many traditional medicines, increasing this newfound interest. Herbal medicine is getting back into the limelight, rejuvenated by new research findings, digital platforms spreading knowl-edge, and a worldwide community of passionate practitioners and advocates (Pan et al., 2014; *The History of Herbal Medicine*, 2020).

The Living Legacy

As we near the end of this chapter, it's clear that the story of herbal medicine isn't just a series of historical footnotes. It's a dynamic, ever-changing story with countless breakthroughs and much-needed insights. Our journey takes us from the historic Nile to today's state-of-the-art labs, with each effort adding another layer of understanding to how we view and use plants. At its heart, herbalism stays true to its grassroots origins—a body of knowledge lovingly nurtured and handed down through generations. By learning about and using the limitless possibilities of plants, we are making a conscious contribution to our future generations.

Chapter 2

Understanding Plant Power
Basics of Herbal Constituents

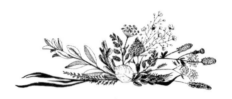

Plants are the young of the world, vessels of health and vigor; but they grope ever upward towards consciousness; the trees are imperfect men, and seem to bemoan their imprisonment, rooted in the ground.

— Ralph Waldo Emerson

Here, we venture into the basics of herbal constituents, discovering the incredible energy and complexity hidden within plants. This chapter highlights some key elements, such as flavonoids, tannins, terpenes, alkaloids, saponins, and phenolic acids. Each section will reveal how these natural components, often unnoticed, significantly contribute to a plant's life and, intriguingly, to our health and well-being.

Did you know that plants can influence everything from our mood and cognitive functions to our digestive, metabolic, and cardiovascular health? More importantly, we'll see how all these elements work together in synergy, which shows us just how interconnected nature truly is.

What Are Phytochemicals?

Strolling through a garden, have you ever considered you're amidst a vast, natural pharmacy? It's a space overflowing with nature's health-boosting agents: phytochemicals. These phytochemicals, nestled quietly within plants, are crucial both for plant vitality and our own health.

Let's explore phytochemicals through everyday experiences: The vibrant reds of tomatoes, the lush blues of berries, and the bright greens of leafy veggies, not to mention the inviting aroma of your morning herbal tea, are all the thanks to phytochemicals. They add a touch of much-needed color, enticing scents, and delicious flavors to our daily meals—can you imagine a world where you no longer taste or smell your favorite dish? Yet, phytochemicals go beyond our sensory pleasure; they are critical to our body's defense and count toward our health.

As we glimpse the spectrum of phytochemicals, we find flavonoids with their antioxidant prowess, protecting cells from aging and illness. Then there are tannins, offering bitter tastes in fruits and wines along with their protective qualities. The variety of phytochemicals is expansive, each contributing uniquely to our health and flavor.

Our meals are opportunities to embrace these tiny but mighty elements. By simply eating a crunchy apple, enjoying a cup of green tea, or adding cinnamon to oatmeal, you're tapping into a wealthy phytochemical source. Every piece of fruit, vegetable, and herb in our diet plays a significant part in our health. Could nature have always intended to nurture our health in such a harmonious way?

Flavonoids

You're enjoying a delicious pear or appreciating a warm cup of tea... Little do you realize that with every bite and sip, you're absorbing various beneficial compounds that champion our health–meet the flavonoids. These phytonutrients don't just splash color across our fruits and veggies; they are the hidden warriors in grains and our gardens.

Flavonoids are like nature's multi-functional toolkit, each meticulously designed to boost our health. Envision them as tiny yet effective protectors, arming our cells with antioxidant defenses, fending off free radicals, and building defensive walls against inflammation, viruses, and cancer (Santos & Silva, 2020). As you indulge in a plump berry or savor a glass of robust red wine, consider these microscopic soldiers diligently safeguarding our health, quietly working to revive our hearts and slow down the aging process.

The different types of flavonoids include:

- **Anthocyanins:** They provide our meals with vibrant reds, purples, and blues, as we can see in berries and grapes, adding not just color but also vitality.
- **Flavones:** Subtle yet significant, they can be found in various herbs and vegetables, also contributing to our wellness.

Furthermore, flavonoids are essential in ensuring our hearts beat consistently and healthily. Similarly, these compounds act as a gentle nudge to our brain cells, enhancing memory and cognitive functions—think of it as your morning coffee.

Tannins

We've all experienced the puckering sensation of an overly steeped tea or the dry mouthfeel after biting into an unripe persimmon. Tannins are responsible for that one-of-a-kind sensation! They make a bold statement wherever they happen to be. These phytochemicals are versatile protectors in the broader domain of plant chemistry and are much more than their bitter taste.

There are two types of tannins:

- **Hydrolyzable tannins:** These are found in oak galls and tea leaves.
- **Condensed tannins:** Commonly present in grapes, wine, and chocolate.

Tannins, often unnoticed, are vital in maintaining the intricate balance found in nature. Also, as a safeguard, they protect us against harmful microbes and viruses, creating challenging environments where these threats can't survive. Not only do they fend off potential pathogens, but they also serve as antioxidants, quietly guarding our cells against oxidative stress—a critical factor in aging and disease prevention (*American Herbal Pharmacopoeia*, 2023). Their antioxidant mastery ensures that our body's processes, including digestion and heart health, remain in excellent condition.

Now, let's connect some dots. The slight bitterness in your tea, perhaps your glass of red wine, or the durability of your leather jacket? That's tannins working their magic. They've enriched our history, being essential in traditional medicines for wound healing and inflammation, giving our food a unique edge, and even playing a crucial role in the leather industry. So, with tannins adding depth to both our palates and healthiness, it makes us wonder: What other plant-based wonders are subtly enhancing our daily lives?

Terpenes

Envision yourself entering a forest where the aromas of fresh pine, calming lavender, and energizing citrus zest mix harmoniously with each breath you take. That's what the terpenes are for; consider them nature's own fragrance experts! These aromatic compounds are actively involved in the field of health and well-being, along with offering us stunning scents in the air.

They take on roles like reducing inflammation, soothing pain, and fighting against bacterial and fungal adversaries. These compounds have tangible effects on our mood and stress levels, too! Consider the calmness that a lavender-scented bath offers after a long day or the refreshing sensation of peeling an orange —evidence of terpenes at work.

These small compounds in plants, such as sage, peppermint, and chamomile, go beyond their aromatic characteristics. They delve into complex health science areas, including their intriguing yet slightly evasive role in mediating estrogenic effects through alpha estrogen receptors (Canivenc-Lavier & Bennetau-Pelissero, 2023).

In both traditional and modern medicine, plants rich in these estrogen-mimicking terpenes are gaining more attention. More research is being done on its potential role in managing hormonal cancers, alleviating menopausal symptoms, and possibly influencing cardiovascular, immune, and inflammatory conditions. Terpenes in plants like clary sage, chamomile, and niaouli are often refined into concentrated essential oils, the very ones we use at home in our diffusers, to create a calming space while you go about your day.

Anethole, a standout in this group, found in fennel, star anise, and cumin, is notable for its traditional use in soothing digestion, easing premenstrual discomfort, and improving lactation. This illustrates how terpenes aren't just playing with our sense of smell; they're engaging in a kind of aromatic enchantment, weaving their magic into our health and daily lives. With their widespread influence, terpenes remind us there's always more to discover in the fascinating world of plant-based compounds.

Alkaloids

Alkaloids are the sharp-tongued members of the phytochemical family; much like tannins, they are often associated with a bitter taste. They are found in coffee, tea, and certain medicinal herbs; alkaloids such as caffeine, quinine, and morphine are renowned for their influential pharmacological effects. They've been used in medicine for their pain-relieving, anti-malaria, and stimulant properties. However, it's their dual nature–helpful in appropriate amounts and potentially harmful in excess– that reminds us of the importance of respecting and understanding natural compounds.

Saponins

Saponins may fly under the radar compared to other phytochemicals, but their roles are crucial and increasingly recognized. These compounds, famous for their soap-like foaminess in water, appear in our everyday eats like beans, quinoa, and ginseng. Saponins are more than simply nature's cleansers; they also have some highly effective health-promoting properties. Their potential to improve immunity and lower cholesterol has drawn the attention of experts and health enthusiasts alike.

But that's just scratching the surface. These multitaskers are known for playing defense and protecting plants from pesky invaders like insects and microbes. What's more, these compounds are turning heads in the commercial world. Their unique combination of structural properties—a blend of a triterpene or steroid core with sugar chains—makes them notable not just in the health sphere but also in food, cosmetics, and pharmaceuticals.

Thanks to growing consumer interest in all things natural, along with their surfactant qualities—think natural soap—saponins are stepping into the spotlight in various industries. They're more than an unexplored ingredient; they represent a gateway to innovative applications. Yet, their complex nature presents challenges in processing ways to extract and purify them. Luckily, there is more research on the rise that not only sheds light on the sources and properties of saponins but also focuses on the nitty-gritty of their extraction, purification, and how processing impacts their structure and benefits. Saponins aren't just about making bubbles; they're emerging as dynamic participants searching for healthier, more natural product choices.

Phenolic Acids

Despite receiving less attention, phenolic acids are widely present in fruits, vegetables, grains, nuts, seeds, and nuts. They serve as fantastic antioxidants essential in preventing oxidative stress and related illnesses. Not only do they appear to have anti-inflammatory properties, but they may also help prevent long-term health issues, including diabetes and heart disease.

How Plants Affect the Human Body

The way plants interact with our bodies is truly incredible! It's like a magical embrace of complexity and effectiveness. As we know, aside from their nutritional significance, plant compounds can have a significant impact on our body's functioning, health, and overall well-being. But just how deep does it go? Let's have a look below.

Mood and Cognition

Just as a soothing cup of chamomile tea can calm our nerves, other remarkable herbs like Rhodiola rosea and ashwagandha have the ability to tweak our brain functions. These herbs contain adaptogens, which are the natural agents that help our bodies counter various stressors, whether physical, chemical, or biological. Rhodiola, well-known for its stress-buffering adaptogenic qualities, is essential in enhancing our mood and ensuring mental clarity and cognitive function. It regulates the body's stress responses, combats fatigue, and has been found effective in clinical trials for improving mood, reducing anxiety, and enhancing overall cognitive performance, especially under stress (Adaes, 2018; Güçlü-Üstündağ & Mazza, 2023).

Similarly, ashwagandha, another potent adaptogen, has shown impressive results in easing perimenopausal symptoms in women, significantly easing psychological, somatic-vegetative, and urogenital discomforts while positively affecting their hormonal balances (Gopal et al., 2021). This herbal duo underlines the potential of natural adaptogens to boost our mental well-being and cognitive resilience.

The Green Glow

Digestive and Metabolic Health

Traditionally cherished herbs like peppermint, ginger, and fennel are known to relieve our stomach discomforts. But did you know these herbs and others like turmeric and cinnamon do more than just taste good? A recent study by Champagne et al. (2019) explored plant phytochemicals and their role in resistance against herbivores, suggesting potential health benefits for us, too. Phenolics, found in herbs like turmeric, show anti-inflammatory and antioxidant properties, which could be game-changers in tackling conditions like diabetes and obesity. Likewise, the terpenes in ginger and peppermint, which once defended plants against hungry critters, could be our best allies in digestive health. So next time you sprinkle some cinnamon or sip on peppermint tea, remember—Mother Nature is doing her thing without us having to try!

Cardiovascular Health

Flavonoid-rich plants, such as hawthorn and garlic, support cardiovascular well-being. They contribute to blood pressure modulation, help with lowering our cholesterol, and prevent our arteries from blockage. Similarly, herbs like green tea are a source of catechins, compounds Ruskovska et al. (2020) found to enhance blood circulation and decrease cholesterol levels. This study also revealed the subtle gene-regulatory effects of flavanols, such as those in green tea, highlighting their role in inflammation and lipid metabolism. The growing understanding of these molecular mechanisms can potentially guide us toward better-tailored nutritional advice in the future. In the meantime, enjoy your green tea!

The Harmony of Synergy in Plant-Based Compounds

In exploring the world of plant-based compounds, we're not just looking at individual elements but at how they work together to create effects far greater than the sum of their parts. Think of a plant as a complex puzzle. Each nutrient is a piece on its own impressive, but when combined, they create a stunning image that not only delights our senses but also helps boost our well-being.

Here are two examples of how nature collaborates to bring us the best of both worlds:

- **Green tea:** More than just a soothing drink, green tea is a prime example of synergy. Its catechins, or the powerful antioxidants, work with natural caffeine to provide a gentle, lasting energy uplift, contrasting the sharp kick we receive from our cup of coffee.
- **Turmeric and black pepper:** This duo is a synergy masterpiece. Curcumin in turmeric, enhanced by piperine in black pepper, increases curcumin's absorption, amplifying its joint anti-inflammatory properties. So, feel free to sprinkle it generously!

But how does this synergy work? Certain plant compound combinations can significantly boost our body's ability to absorb and use these nutrients. These phytochemicals address various health aspects or pathways, providing a broad and practical approach to help prevent and treat multiple conditions. It's like amplifying the health effects by knowing what works well together. In both traditional herbal medicine and age-old healing practices, the concept of synergy is vital.

So, if you want to add some of this magic to your own herbal practice, opt for whole plant extracts instead of isolated compounds that can capture the full range of a plant's healing abilities. Many health practitioners take years to customize their treatments; it takes time to develop precise and effective remedies, so be patient with yourself.

Grasping the concept of synergy in plants goes further than simply appreciating nature's complexity; it involves integrating this knowledge into how we manage our health. The collaboration among various plant compounds, such as antioxidants, vitamins, and minerals, represents a more unified approach to health, recognizing each component's vital role within a broader wellness context. As our understanding of plant chemistry expands, it can transform our health perspectives, directing us to align closer with the refined patterns found in nature. This philosophy isn't only intriguing; it's essential in redefining how we use our plants for health, highlighting the importance of seeing them as a holistic, interconnected network.

Chapter 3

Growing Your Own Green Pharmacy

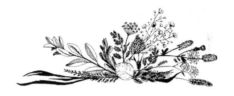

The love of gardening is a seed once sown that never dies.

— Gertrude Jekyll.

This is the chapter for cultivating green thumbs and nurturing curious minds! We can't deny the magic when we see a tiny seed grow into a lush green source of healing (plant power, am I right?). When we know how to grow our own herbs, it's about more than having fresh garnishing on hand for pasta night or to impress the dinner guests; it's about taking charge of our health and staying connected to nature.

So, get ready to set up your garden space, learn how to care for your herbs, which herbs you can quickly start off with, and a few more tips and tricks to help your plants thrive no matter the season. Let's get growing!

Setting Up Your Herb Garden

The joys of creating an herbal haven right in your backyard or on your windowsill! But first, we must ensure we choose the right space and use suitable soil. Here's how you know what is right for your garden (DeJohn, 2023):

Selecting the Right Spot

Essential factors to consider as you choose where to grow your plants:

- **Sunlight:** Most herbs enjoy full sun, which means they need at least 6–8 hours of sunlight daily. Keep an eye on your potential garden spots during the day to see which areas receive good sunlight. However, some herbs, like mint and parsley, like cool shaded spots.
- **Proximity to the house:** For ease, it's a good idea to place your garden near your kitchen or back door. This allows easy access when you need fresh herbs for cooking—think rosemary with the roast or fresh basil pesto paninis!
- **Drainage:** Make sure your space doesn't accumulate water after a rainy day. Herbs don't like "wet feet," meaning they don't thrive in waterlogged soil, so avoid forming mini ponds. Elevated beds or sloped areas usually provide better drainage.

Using the Right Soil

Some things to consider when it comes to the type of soil as you get ready to plant:

- **Soil types:** Herbs generally prefer well-draining soil with a pH level between 6.0 and 7.5. What would the ideal mix be? Loamy soil! It is a balanced mix of sand, silt, and clay. However, many herbs can tolerate various soil types if the water drains well.
- **Soil testing:** Before planting, consider testing your soil! There are many soil testing kits available at garden centers or online stores such as Amazon. It's a neat way to know your soil's secrets—like its pH and nutrient levels—and give your herbs precisely what they need.
- **Soil amendment:** Based on your soil test results, you might need to tweak your soil (*Rodale Institute*, 2021). For increasing drainage, you might consider adding organic compost or well-decomposed manure. To adjust the pH, you can use lime to raise the pH or sulfur to lower the pH.

City Garden Scapes

So, you might not have much backyard to grow your dream garden, and that's okay, too! Below are guidelines on how to grow a garden despite living in an urban area:

- **Limited space:** For those with space limitations, vertical gardening can be a game-changer. Use wall-mounted planters, one-of-a-kind hanging pots, or stylish trellises to maximize that vertical space.
- **Poor soil quality:** In urban areas, the existing soil might be degraded or of poor quality. Using raised beds with store-bought potting mix can create a more controlled environment for your herbs.

- **Balcony or window sills:** For apartment dwellers, balcony or windowsill gardens can be quite valuable! Always be sure to choose containers with good drainage and place them in areas that receive good sunlight, and you'll revel in green goodness in no time!

The main thing to take away from this section? Observe, adapt, and have fun along the way!

Basics of Planting, Nurturing, and Harvesting Medicinal Plants

So, you chose your spot, and you have the soil ready; now what? We plant, we nurture, and we harvest! Here is an essential step-by-step guide on how to take care of your new herb garden (Moss, 2023; *National Gardening Association*, 2023):

Planting

This seems obvious, but important nonetheless! Keep the following in mind as you plant your herbs:

- **Seeding:** Begin by selecting high-quality seeds from trusted sources. Some medicinal plants can also be propagated from cuttings or root divisions. Prepare a loose, well-draining soil mix, and plant the seeds or cuttings at the depth the plant prefers, as each species has a different liking.
- **Spacing:** Give them room to breathe! Ensure adequate spacing between plants to prevent overcrowding and stimulate air circulation, reducing the risk of fungal diseases.

Nurturing

Much like humans, our plants need some TLC, too. How can we show our plants love and care? By nurturing each species on their own terms. Below are all-around guidelines to consider:

- **Watering:** Medicinal plants, like all plants, need water, but the quantity and frequency will vary. Too much? They're flooded. Too little? They're parched. Over-watering can lead to root rot while under-watering can stress the plant. As a general rule, water them when the top inch of the soil feels dry. Aim for moist, not swampy.
- **Pruning:** Give your plants a slight trim now and then. By regularly pruning your plants, you encourage healthy growth! Remove any dead (droopy) or yellowing leaves and spent flowers. This not only improves their appearance but also redirects their energy to sprouting new growth.
- **Pest control:** Opt for organic pest control methods that are safe and eco-friendly. Natural options like neem oil, soapy solutions, and beneficial (plant-friendly) insects like ladybugs can help chase away common pests. Regularly check your plants for signs of uninvited critters and address these issues promptly.

Harvesting

Let's be honest; this is what we've all been waiting for: the harvest of our lush green growth! But let's not just take it greedily; we need to be mindful as we gather:

- **Leaves:** Have you ever wondered when to pluck those leaves? Right before the flower show begins! The best time to harvest leaves is just before the plant flowers when they have the highest concentration of active compounds. Cut leaves in the early morning as this is prime time, right after the dew has evaporated, but before the sun becomes too intense.

- **Roots:** Autumn is usually the best time to harvest roots, as the plant has stored energy in them throughout the summer. Gently unearth the plant, shake off the soil, and rinse the roots thoroughly.
- **Flowers:** Pick flowers as they open—hello, world! Again, early morning is optimal after the dew has dried before the midday sun. This ensures they keep their essential oils, contributing to their magical medicinal properties.
- **Maximizing potency:** To maintain the potency of the plant's harvested parts, dry them promptly. Spread them in a single layer on a suitable surface, such as a tray in a well-ventilated (breezy) area away from direct sunlight. Store dried materials in airtight containers, away from light and heat.
- **Shelf-life:** Properly dried and stored medicinal plant materials can last a year or more, but their potency decreases over time because, like fine wine, herbs age. It's a good idea to label containers with the date of harvest and use older stock first.

What a journey! The art of growing medicinal plants is filled with love and patience. Pay close attention to your planting, nurturing, and harvesting practices to ensure your plants offer the most therapeutic benefits. By being attentive and hands-on, you'll have a thriving green garden in no time—here's to your health and vitality!

Easy-to-Grow Herbs for Beginners

The world of herbs is expansive, and the list of species is simply overwhelming, especially for newer green thumbs, so below, you will discover a handful of beginner-friendly medicinal herbs (*Herbal Encyclopedia*, 2010; Neveln, 2016):

Mint (Mentha)

- **Cultivation needs:** Mint is a versatile plant, happy in partial shade and even in full sun. It thrives in well-draining soil and requires regular watering. Be cautious, as mint can be invasive; consider planting it in containers to keep it from taking over your garden.
- **Medicinal properties:** Mint is well-known for its digestive benefits. It can help soothe stomachaches, reduce gas, and is a natural remedy for nausea.
- **Home use:** Are you a regular tea drinker? Add mint! The leaves can also be added to salads, juices, or desserts for a minty flavor.

Basil (Ocimum basilicum)

- **Cultivation needs:** Basil loves full sun and thrives in moist, well-drained soil. Regularly pinch the stems to keep your plant full and delay flowering, giving flavorful leaves.
- **Medicinal properties:** While commonly recognized for its culinary uses, basil has anti-inflammatory properties and benefits our digestive health.
- **Home use:** Known as the star ingredient in pesto, basil can be used in many dishes, bringing a fresh, aromatic

flavor. Try different varieties for a twist–some offer
hints of lemon, anise, or even cinnamon!

Lavender (Lavandula)

- **Cultivation needs:** Lavender needs full sun and well-
  draining, with slightly alkaline soil. It's drought-
  tolerant and doesn't like to be overwatered—don't
  drown them!
- **Medicinal properties:** Need to unwind and relax?
  Known for its relaxing and anxiety-reducing effects. It
  can also help alleviate headaches and improve sleep
  quality.
- **Home use:** Dried lavender buds can be added to
  sachets and placed in drawers or under your pillows to
  encourage relaxation. Lavender essential oils can be
  used for aromatherapy (a few essential oil drops in the
  diffuser ensure a restful night's sleep) or diluted for
  topical application.

Chives (Allium schoenoprasum)

- **Cultivation needs:** Chives also enjoy a spot with full
  sun to partial shade and prefer their soil moist and
  well-drained.
- **Medicinal properties:** Beyond their delicate onion
  flavor, chives are rich in vitamins and minerals,
  including vitamin K and manganese.
- **Home use:** Sprinkle them onto dishes for a mild,
  onion-like flavor. Guess what? Their pinkish-purple
  flowers are not only attractive but are also edible and
  can add beauty and taste to our salads!

Cilantro (Coriandrum sativum)

- **Cultivation needs:** This herb prefers cool weather, blooming as temperatures rise. Ensure it's planted in well-draining soil and gets plenty of sun.
- **Medicinal properties:** Cilantro is known to be rich in antioxidants and may help support our heart health.
- **Home use:** Widely used in Mexican and Asian cuisines, the fresh leaves bring a unique flavor. Some might find it unpalatable, while others can't get enough. Bonus? The seeds of this plant are known as coriander, a popular spice used in various dishes.

Fennel (Foeniculum vulgare)

- **Cultivation needs:** Fennel craves full sunlight and thrives in moist, well-drained soil.
- **Medicinal properties:** It has been used as a remedy for digestive issues, including heartburn, bloating, and loss of appetite.
- **Home use:** The nutty, anise-like flavor of fennel is welcomed into various dishes. And we can use the whole plant when cooking, as both its bulb and seeds are edible.

Lemon Balm (Melissa officinalis)

- **Cultivation needs:** Preferring a spot with either full sun or part shade, lemon balm flourishes in moist, well-draining soil.
- **Medicinal properties:** Lemon balm has a calming effect and can help relieve symptoms of anxiety or insomnia.

- **Home use:** Steep the fragrant leaves in hot water for a soothing herbal tea, or add them to dishes for a citrusy flavor; you might just pleasantly surprise your guests with a hint of citrus in your next salad.

Parsley (Petroselinum crispum)

- **Cultivation needs:** This easy-to-grow herb enjoys full sun to partial shade and moist, well-drained soil.
- **Medicinal properties:** Rich in vitamins, especially vitamin C, parsley is not just a garnish but a health booster! The more, the better.
- **Home use:** Add chopped parsley to elevate the flavors in your dishes, or use the curly variety to decorate your dinner plates.

Rosemary (Rosmarinus officinalis)

- **Cultivation needs:** Favoring full sunlight, rosemary needs well-draining soil and doesn't like to sit in water; do not overwater this variety.
- **Medicinal properties:** Known to improve our concentration, rosemary also has anti-inflammatory benefits.
- **Home use:** Their aromatic leaves are perfect for flavoring meats and vegetables. Try adding it to your bread dough; if you're feeling Greek, infuse your extra virgin olive oil with a sprig or two.

Thyme (Thymus vulgaris)

- **Cultivation needs:** Thyme loves full sun and prefers light, well-draining soil.

- **Medicinal properties:** This plant is known for its antibacterial properties and can help with respiratory issues—so you can just breathe.
- **Home use:** Infuse your dishes with the intense, earthy aroma of thyme, either fresh or dried. It pairs beautifully with meats and roasted vegetables.

Thus, in essence, these herbs are ideal for beginners like yourself and have a ton of health benefits. Enjoy the satisfaction of knowing that the medicinal plants you've worked so hard to nurture and develop are coming fresh from your own garden.

Seasonal Tips for Herb Cultivation

As with all things in life, herbs change with the seasons. Your question, then, is, how do you keep them thriving all year long? Let's have a look at what each season brings (Richter, 2023):

Spring

- **Planting:** As the last frost disappears, it's the ideal time to plant most herbs. Seeds or young plants can be introduced to well-prepared beds that have premium soil.
- **Fertilization:** Add a light, balanced fertilizer to help jump-start their growth after the more dormant winter months.
- **Pruning:** Spring is also the prime time for pruning. Cut back any dead stems from the previous year to make way for new, vibrant growth.

Summer

- **Watering:** Hydrate to keep them glowing and growing! The summer heat means your herbs will need more frequent watering. However, avoid over-watering, as you don't want them to be soggy.
- **Harvesting:** This is it! It's time to pick those stunning greens. Summer is the peak harvesting time for most herbs. Always harvest in the morning for the best flavor, and be sure you never take more than one-third of the plant; they need some leaves to keep doing their thing.

Autumn

- **Preparing for winter:** As cooler temperatures start rolling in, it's time to provide them with some snug, so consider putting mulch around your herbs to provide that insulation (Iannotti, 2022). If you have perennial herbs, trim them to encourage more vigorous growth in spring.
- **Transition them indoors:** If you live in an area with harsh winters, consider moving some of your herbs to pots and bringing them indoors. They'll appreciate the indoor warmth.

Winter

- **Indoor care:** Herbs inside need a sunny spot; your window should be perfect; remember to water them sparingly. Ensure good air circulation by opening a window for fresh air and to prevent mold from forming.

- **Protection:** For outdoor perennial herbs, provide extra love and keep them well-mulched. Some, like rosemary, may need more protection, like a burlap wrap in areas with severe frost.

General Tips for Changing Seasons

- **Indoor vs. outdoor:** If you're transferring plants indoors or out with the changing seasons, don't rush the process; rather, acclimate them gradually. Start by placing them in their new environment for a few hours each day, slowly increasing the time spent in their new space.
- **Weather watch:** Always watch the forecast, as Mother Nature can be unpredictable. A sudden frost or scorching day, in particular, heatwaves, can catch us off guard, so be ready with things like frost cloths or shade nets to keep your herbs thriving.

In this chapter, we've had the pleasure of looking into the incredible world of gardening and the many benefits it brings. From getting your space ready to the excitement of harvesting, every step teaches us the importance of patience, taking care, and appreciating our close connection with nature. As you start your gardening journey, take your time, learn as you go, and, most importantly, have fun along the way! Happy gardening to you!

Chapter 4

Herbal Teas

Sips of Wellness

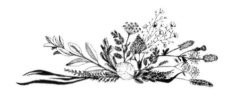

There is something in the nature of tea that leads us into a world of quiet contemplation of life.

— Lin Yutang

Welcome to the comfy corner of Chapter 4! Here, we'll explore the vibrant world of herbal brews—a wealth of vibrancy in every cup. With every leaf and root infused in hot water, a simple sip can be a source of healing joy and bring us closer to the wonders of nature.

We'll discover the benefits of herbal beverages outside the traditional tea leaf, turning every cup into a personal health remedy and a soothing ritual. We'll even make our herbal blends! Get ready to discover the world of herbal teas and how they can add to our daily dose of well-being.

The Essence of Herbal Teas

Discover the aromatic world of herbal teas and experience a legacy that is both ageless and wholesome (*The Herb Guide*, 2023). These are more than simply teas—consider the many combinations of leaves, flowers, seeds, and roots that give benefits beyond the flavor. Every cup connects us to a history of healers who have harnessed the life-sustaining power of plants, stretching from ancient cultures to modern health enthusiasts. Consider mint, which energizes; chamomile, which calms; and echinacea, which protects us like our own plant bodyguard!

Brewing the Perfect Cup: An Art and Science

Now, let's talk about crafting that perfect cup of herbal tea—a blend of intuition and precision, a gentle process where art and science meet right in your kitchen!

Here's how to make magic with your herbal teas (*TeaUSA*, 2013):

- **Water:** Begin with the most purified water; filtered or spring water is best. Tap water will do if it's not too alkaline.
- **Your chosen herb:** Place your chosen herbs in a teapot or infuser. Loose leaves prefer space to expand and release their full potential; they're quite the free spirits.
- **Temperature:** Each herb has its own favored temperature. Tender buds and petals like a soft heat, somewhere between 160 and 180 °F, while the hardy roots and barks are all about the heat and can endure up to 212 °F.

- **Timing is everything:** The steeping time sets the rhythm for your tea's flavor; a quick 3–5 minutes usually hits the mark, but if you're after a more full-bodied taste, feel free to steep up to 10 minutes.
- **Storage them safely:** To keep your herbs vibrant and compelling, store them in airtight containers away from light and warmth; a dark pantry or cupboard is perfect.

If you want to experiment, you are welcome to do so! The rules of brewing the perfect pot are not set in stone, so adjust the times and temperatures as you find what works for you.

Here is guidance on how to tailor your next brew:

- **Customize the strength:** Want a stronger sip? For a more robust flavor, add more herbs, but remember, steeping it for too long might make it bitter.
- **For the sweet tooth:** If you're after a touch of sweetness, honey or stevia are your go-to companions —they'll harmonize with your brew without overpowering it.
- **Fresh citrus:** A splash of lemon or orange peel can elevate the lighter notes of your tea and add some fresh summer tones!
- **Cold brew:** For those who favor a chilled sip, let your mixture mingle in cold water in the refrigerator overnight. It offers a gentle approach for a mellow taste.
- **Adding milk:** Milk or a dairy-free alternative can provide your tea with creamy luxury, perfect for taming bolder infusions into a silky-smooth experience.

Remember, adventurous tea blenders, that each cup is your own custom-made elixir, and there is a certain amount of satisfaction in identifying the blend designed especially for you. Dare to combine flavor with ease, allowing each cup to honor both your creativity and respected tradition.

The Herbal Tea Pantry: Our Essentials for Wellness

Let's enter the herbal tea pantry, where delicious flavors and well-being go hand-in-hand. In the world of herbal teas, there are plenty! So here is a list with a few notable ones to know about (Jones, 2017; Wack, 2021):

- **Chamomile:** Think of chamomile as a gentle caress for your senses. With subtle floral hints and a soft golden hue, this herb is a lullaby in a cup, perfect for easing into a peaceful sleep.
- **Peppermint:** This one's the life of the party in the tea world, with its invigorating scent and a refreshing taste that wakes up our taste buds! It's a go-to for soothing an upset stomach.
- **Lavender:** A sip of lavender tea is like strolling through a field of purple flowers somewhere in the South of France! It's a calming source for those restless nights and a go-to for soothing stress.
- **Ginger:** Bold and spicy, ginger brings a warming zest perfect for digestion and energizing our senses! Simmer some freshly sliced ginger for a strong brew that ignites good health.
- **Echinacea:** Gentle floral notes with a touch of zest, echinacea is like a shield for our immune systems. Just

a short infusion period is enough to prepare this fortifying drink.

- **Hibiscus:** Hibiscus blooms give your cup a ruby-red color and a tart flavor full of vitality and vitamins.
- **Rosehip:** Rich in vitamin C and friendly to your skin, the subtle, fruity charm of rosehip makes a rejuvenating tea that's beauty in a cup.
- **Nettle:** This underrated herb is a nutritional powerhouse, dense with minerals, and supports our overall health. Once simmered, it transforms into a deeply nourishing beverage.
- **Licorice root:** Naturally sweet and comforting, licorice root brings a smooth, soothing quality to any blend, perfect for calming a sore throat and easing anxiety.
- **Dandelion root:** Beyond its reputation as a stubborn weed, the dandelion's root is a detoxifying ally, supporting our liver function.
- **Tulsi (holy basil):** Sacred in many traditions, tulsi's unique flavor is at the heart of many restorative teas.
- **Cinnamon:** This familiar spice brings warmth and a hint of sweetness, promoting digestion and adding a cozy note to any tea blend.
- **Cardamom:** Fragrant and slightly spicy, cardamom pods infuse a distinctive, therapeutic flavor.
- **Butterfly pea flower:** With a vibrant blue hue, this tea is high in antioxidants and has anti-inflammatory and cognitive benefits.
- **Rooibos:** Grown in South African bushes, caffeine-free rooibos is packed with antioxidants and is excellent for our heart health.

- **Lemongrass:** This citrusy herb balances digestive health, antimicrobial properties, and anxiety alleviation in a refreshing method.
- **Cota (Navajo tea):** An indigenous brew with earthy notes, Cota comforts the digestive system with its gentle touch.

Embrace these herbal heroes in your tea pantry, and you'll not only craft cups of comfort but also brew well-being into each day. Experiment with delight, sip with intent, and watch your wellness garden grow one cup at a time.

Creating Your Own Blends

This is the space where you can be creative. It's all about mixing and matching, finding the perfect matches in flavor and function (*American Herbalists Guild*, 2013):

- **Flavor fusion:** Each herb has a flavor profile—mint is cooling, cinnamon is warming, chamomile is soothing, and so on. Learning the basic profiles will serve as your guide to blending. You want to achieve a harmony where no herb overpowers the other unless that's what you want. Consider how the flavors will interact. Some flavors naturally click, such as mint and lemon, while others bring out the best in each other when paired, like rose and hibiscus, for example. Start with a foundation—mild green tea or the ever-versatile rooibos—then introduce a complementary note such as a zesty citrus or a sweet berry, and then a final touch for that extra tang, consider adding a sprinkle of cinnamon or a slice of ginger.

- **Combining for wellness:** Have you considered tailoring your tea to your wellness goals? Decide what the goal of your tea is. For relaxation, you might focus on herbs like lavender, chamomile, and lemon balm. For a digestive aid, peppermint, ginger, and fennel might be your go-to.
- **Getting the ratio right:** When creating a blend, a beginner-friendly method uses three parts of your base herb, one part of a complementary herb, and one of an accent herb. This isn't a strict rule but rather a starting point! The "base" is usually the dominant flavor or the herb with the preferred primary effect. The "complementary" adds depth and supports the primary function, while the "accent" introduces a contrasting note, often for a touch of complexity or a hint of sharpness to elevate the overall blend. Don't be afraid to try odd pairings! For example, a base of green tea might be enhanced with the floral notes of rose petals as a complement and a pinch of black pepper as an accent for an unexpected kick.

Here are recipes to get you started at home (*Simple Loose Leaf Tea Company*, 2020):

Lemon and Elderflower Tea

This blend is perfect for those looking to combat the symptoms of the common cold (goodbye sniffles)!

Blend the following for one cup:

- 1 tablespoon of elderflowers—fresh or dried
- 1–2 teaspoons of lemon juice
- 1 teaspoon of honey

Classic Cinnamon and Apple Tea

A timeless herbal fruit tea blend that's incredibly cozy in cooler weather.

The following is enough for one cup:

- 1 tablespoon of dried apple pieces
- ½ tablespoon of crushed cinnamon bark

Chamomile and Lemon Balm Sleep Tea

Are you struggling to fall asleep at night, and lavender just doesn't do the trick? Try this combination!

Blend these ingredients for 3–4 cups:

- 1 tablespoon of dried chamomile flowers
- 1 tablespoon of dried and crushed lemon balm leaves

With each creation, you learn more about the herbs and how they relate to your body and palate. Whether seeking comfort, health, or simply the pleasure of a delicious cuppa, your tea blends provide a more mindful, enhanced tea experience.

Safety and Precautions

Now, before you unleash your inner herbalist, let's talk safety—ensure your tea blending is not just creative but also smart and safe (*American Herbalists Guild*, 2013):

- **Herb-drug interactions:** Some herbs might not mix well with prescription drugs. For instance, St. John's Wort is a known no-match for blood thinners. Always be sure to check with your healthcare professional before mixing herbs into your daily diet or regimen.

- **Allergy awareness:** Like any new food, herbs can sometimes cause adverse reactions. So, introduce new herbs slowly, monitor your body's response, and listen to any warnings it gives.
- **Pregnancy considerations:** If you're expecting, it's wise to exercise extra caution. Some herbs are not recommended during pregnancy, so when in doubt, it's best to err on the side of caution.

For peace of mind, always keep the lines of communication open with your healthcare practitioner. To guarantee that your tea blending experience is delightful and risk-free, taking a few simple precautions may go a long way. Now that you have these suggestions have fun making your own personal tea blends!

Embracing Herbal Teas in Daily Life

As we reach the end of this chapter, like the last soothing sips of your favorite infusion, we're wrapped up in the cozy glimmer of new wisdom. This section has been an open door to delight in a cup that's both a nod to age-old customs and your health. We've gone through the mysteries of herbal blends, and now, with a clear understanding of each plant's profile, you're ready to craft your own herbal combinations. May your cup brim with joy and your heart with peace as you savor your tea.

Chapter 5

Beyond Teas

Other Ways to Use Herbs

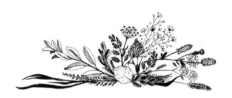

It is my body, my health, my balance, and my responsibility to make the right choices for myself. Right choices include working with competent health-care professionals when necessary, allowing friends and family to help as needed, and, above all, being true to my beliefs, with the wisdom and willingness to change as part of the path of healing.

— Rosemary Gladstar

Think of your favorite tea—maybe it's that peppermint blend that warms you up after a chilly afternoon or the chamomile that's a standby when you need to wind down. Now, imagine stepping out of your comfort zone and into a world where those same herbs can do so much more!

In this chapter, we're not just steeping leaves; we're transforming herbs into a whole cabinet of healing tools. It's like turning your kitchen into a mini lab, but way more fun and without the need for white coats or safety goggles. You'll gently simmer a salve that could soothe your sunburn or the meticulous drip of a tincture tailor-made to ease your friend's relent-less allergies. We're about to get hands-on with some of the most incredible, practical DIY herbal magic (yes, magic—because sometimes it feels pretty close to it when that home-made lip balm works wonders). Here's to the excitement of turning what you've grown or bought into your very own line of personal care products. Let's get started, shall we?

Herbal Prospects: Tinctures, Salves, and More

Who knew that your humble herb collection could do so much? Well, the trusty plants that flavor your tea can also be the heroes in various other healthful concoctions. In this part of the chapter, we'll show the practical and somewhat enchanting process of turning your herbal allies into different preparations—each with its unique charm and specific use (Chappell, 2019; Fletcher, 2019).

Tinctures

Imagine capturing the essence of your garden's vitality in just a few drops. That's the essence of a tincture! These herbal power-houses are created by submerging finely chopped herbs in alcohol or vinegar, releasing their full-bodied benefits into a concentrated extract. After several weeks, once you strain the herbs, you're left with a pure shelf-essence. Their ideal for preserving those delicate plant compounds we've come to cher-ish, tinctures provide us with wellness in each drop, whether it's to support our digestive health or to calm a restless mind.

Salves

When your skin yearns for relief, turn to salves—the herbal world's soothing embrace. By infusing oils with the healing properties of herbs and setting the mixture with beeswax, you create a spreadable, protective balm. Whether it's for a stubborn scar or a bothersome bug bite, salves are an excellent direct application of nature's care. Plus, getting crafty with your own salves allows you to control the consistency and therapeutic properties. Don't forget to perform a patch test with your home-made salve to make sure your skin is compatible.

Poultices

Poultices are the time-honored tradition of applying raw herbs directly to the skin, a practice that invites the healing energy of nature to address our areas of concern. Whether it's a mash of freshly picked plantain for a bee sting or a warm chamomile paste to soothe those sore muscles after a straining workout, poultices offer us direct relief by combining the raw qualities of herbs with the body's own healing mechanisms. Keep your poultices simple and fresh, and use them to complement your body's natural healing processes.

Infused Oils

The alchemy of transforming herbs into infused oils is a gentle process of coaxing out the lipid-soluble constituents. Whether it's lavender for relaxation or arnica for bruises, these oils become the foundation for many herbal products. Preparing your own means, you can choose the strength and scent, tailoring them to your needs or desires. When creating your infusions, choose a high-quality carrier oil and let the mixture steep in a warm, sunny spot to maximize those herbal benefits.

Herbal Vinegar

Herbal vinegars might be the most versatile performers in your herbal lineup. More than a tangy addition to salads, they're a medium for wellness, rich in minerals, and perfect as a digestive aid or a heart-healthy tonic. Keen to try it at home? Infuse apple cider vinegar with herbs like dandelion or nettle, and you'll have a tonic that's as delicious as it is beneficial. Start with a simple recipe, and experiment with different herbs to find the flavor profiles and health benefits that serve you best.

Hopefully, this section inspired you to explore the various uses of herbs! With each creation, you'll become more adept at transforming your greens into something that fits your lifestyle. So, here's to the craft of herbal preparation—equal parts science, intuition, and a dash of intuitive charm.

Basic DIY Herbal Recipes for Common Ailments

In this section, we'll explore some foundational recipes that transform everyday herbs into influential allies against everyday ailments. From relaxing minor discomforts to freeing you from stress, these DIY recipes are designed to be accessible and effective for any budding herbalist (*Healthline*, 2017; *Rosemary Gladstar's Science & Art of Herbalism*, 2016).

Herbal Tincture for Digestive Health

Are you having some stomach discomfort? This tincture might do the trick. Take 1–2 teaspoons of the tincture before meals to help digestion.

Ingredients:

- 1 part dried peppermint leaves
- 1 part dried fennel seeds
- 1 part dried ginger root
- vodka or apple cider vinegar for an alcohol-free alternative

Instructions:

1. Combine the herbs in a clean glass jar.
2. Fill the jar with vodka or vinegar until the herbs are completely submerged.
3. Seal the jar and store it in a cool, dark place for 4–6 weeks, shaking it daily.
4. After the steeping period, strain the liquid through a cheesecloth or fine mesh and store it in a clean, dark glass bottle.

Gentle Calendula Salve for Skin Irritations

If you need a natural remedy for minor cuts, scrapes, or dry skin areas, apply this calendula salve for a soothing effect.

Ingredients:

- 1 cup calendula-infused oil, which is created by steeping dried calendula petals in a carrier oil like olive or almond oil for 2–4 weeks
- 1/4 cup beeswax pellets

Instructions:

1. Gently melt the beeswax in a double boiler.
2. Once melted, add the calendula-infused oil and stir until well combined.
3. Remove from heat and pour into small, sterilized jars.
4. Let it cool and set before sealing the jars.

The Green Glow

Ginger Poultice for Muscle Aches

You had a tough run or strenuous workout, and you need relief! This ginger poultice does wonders for sore muscles or aches.

Ingredients:

- fresh ginger root
- hot
- a clean cloth or gauze

Instructions:

1. Grate a sufficient amount of fresh ginger root.
2. Soak the grated ginger in hot water for a few minutes.
3. Place the soaked ginger onto the cloth and fold it to make a poultice.
4. Apply the poultice to the affected area for 15–20 minutes.

Chamomile and Lavender Sleep Aid Spray

A restful night's sleep is only a spritz away! Spray this mix onto your pillow and linens before bed to promote relaxation and ensure a good night's sleep.

Ingredients:

- 1 cup distilled water
- 2 tablespoons of dried chamomile flowers
- 2 tablespoons of dried lavender flowers
- spray bottle

Instructions:

1. Boil the distilled water and pour over the chamomile and lavender flowers.
2. Let the mixture steep until it cools down to room temperature.
3. Strain the mixture to remove the flowers.
4. Pour the liquid into a spray bottle and apply as needed before bedtime.

Thyme and Honey Cough Syrup

Feeling the mid-winter sniffles and occasional cough? All you need is one tablespoon of this natural cough syrup.

Ingredients:

- 1/4 cup dried thyme leaves
- 1 cup water
- 1 cup honey

Instructions:

1. Boil the water and pour over the thyme leaves, allowing it to steep until it cools.
2. Strain the thyme leaves and combine the infused water with honey in a saucepan.
3. Heat gently, stirring until the honey and thyme water are well combined.
4. Store the mixture in a clean glass bottle.

Safety First: Precautions in Herbal Preparations

As we've already realized, with blending teas, the natural world demands a thoughtful approach. Let's level up that conversation for the more concentrated forms of herbal magic you're working on within this chapter. While some herbs might seem as harmless as a garden party, remember that when concentrated into tinctures, oils, and salves, their potency magnifies (*Better Health Channel*, 2021).

Here are some safety tips to keep in mind for when you start crafting your own recipes:

- **Precision in dosage:** Consider this your measuring mantra: "Start low, go slow." Precision in dosage is critical, especially when a little goes a long way.
- **Spotting sensitive reactions:** Test a patch of skin or start with a tiny dose and wait to see if your body has any new sensations. Your body's feedback is precious; don't ignore the warning signs.
- **Medication mingle-management:** Medications and herbs can have a complicated relationship. Some enhance each other's effects; others might clash. It's best to introduce them cautiously and under the proper guidance, so if you're feeling unsure, it's best to ask your healthcare provider.
- **Quality and source verification:** Sourcing herbs should be done diligently. The origin, purity, and preparation of your herbs can make or break the safety and efficacy of your remedies.
- **Vulnerable populations:** The very young, the elderly, pregnant and nursing individuals, and those with chronic conditions often need gentler, more considered

herbal approaches. In these cases, extra care isn't optional; it's essential.

- **Keeping remedies fresh:** Your homegrown remedies aren't eternal. They need the right conditions to preserve their potency and still be safe. Ensure proper storage for longevity.
- **Continuous education:** Herbal knowledge isn't stagnant; it grows and evolves. Stay informed and up-to-date. Good practices today might be outdated tomorrow, so stay on your toes and keep learning!

The world of herbal remedies is enchanting, but it comes with responsibilities. Your role as an herbalist is part alchemist, part scientist—measuring, testing, and respecting the knowledge of nature at your fingertips. Handle your herbs and practice with care, and you will flourish!

Multi-purpose Herbs and Their Preparations

Isn't it astonishing how a few plants from your garden or windowsill can turn into a full-scale wellness toolkit? The simplicity of preparing these natural remedies makes them accessible to everyone, from the novice cook to the seasoned herbalist.

Here's how we can create our own home remedies from some everyday versatile herbs with minimal effort (Fletcher, 2019; *Healthline*, 2017):

- **Turmeric:** Blend turmeric powder, water, and black pepper to create a paste that fights off inflammation.

- **Garlic:** Infuse garlic cloves in oil over low heat to make a versatile remedy with powerful antibacterial benefits.
- **Peppermint:** Make peppermint oil by steeping dried, crushed leaves in oil for its digestive and cooling properties.
- **Echinacea:** Prepare a tincture by soaking the herb in alcohol to enhance your immune defense.
- **Ginger:** Simmer slices of ginger root in water to make a soothing tea that can aid digestion and reduce nausea.
- **Cinnamon:** Stir cinnamon sticks in warm water or add powdered cinnamon to dishes for its blood sugar-regulating and antimicrobial effects.
- **Thyme:** Create a thyme infusion by steeping the leaves in hot water, which can be used as a throat gargle for its antiseptic properties.
- **Basil:** Steep fresh basil leaves in hot water to create a tea that may alleviate stress and stomach discomfort.
- **Sage:** Boil sage leaves and let them steep to make a strong infusion that can be used as a mouthwash for its antibacterial properties.
- **Lemon balm:** Combine fresh lemon balm leaves with vodka to create a tincture that could help reduce anxiety and promote sleep.

With these effortless preparations, you can get the significant benefits of these plants right in the comfort of your home. Have fun exploring with them!

Healing Is in Your Hands

This chapter emphasizes the enchanting abilities of herbs in advancing our health and wellness. We now know that herbalism is not limited to teas but can be applied to various practices, such as creating tinctures and salves.

Cultivating self-reliance and celebrating each successful remedy as a personal triumph in exploring natural health is essential. The satisfaction of each small victory fuels your passion for learning and growing as an herbalist. By mixing nature's ingredients, we blend tradition with innovation, science with art, and plants with purpose. You can step forward with confidence, knowing that your healing hands can transform the way you care for yourself and your loved ones. The herbs are ready, the knowledge is set, and the natural, healthy life you desire is yours.

Chapter 6

Integrating Herbalism Into Daily Life

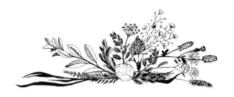

Herbs are the friend of the physician and the pride of cooks.

— Charlemagne

Within the gentle flow of our daily activities, there's an understated yet impactful chance to merge the healing qualities of herbs into our familiar patterns. Herbal practices don't have to be isolated to times of illness or deliberate health pursuits; they can be as routine and constant as the dawn cycle to dusk. This chapter invites you to understand how the ancient knowledge of herbs can seamlessly interact with your day-to-day life, from the aromatic steam of your morning brew to the calming lotion you apply before sleep. Welcome the transition to a lifestyle where your selection of spices also serves as a collection of remedies, and cooking becomes an act of nurturing well-being. Here, we engage in a natural partnership with the environment, welcoming its benefits into our homes, lives, and ordinary experiences. Welcome to the natural inclusion of herbal practices in your life—a journey toward wellness and an enriched bond with the pace of the natural world (Hoshaw, 2021).

Daily Routines With an Herbal Twist

Herbs can be a simple way of improving health and vitality when included in daily routines. The key is to integrate herbal benefits naturally into your day-to-day activities. Below are suggestions for bringing the vitality of herbs into your routine (NT Contributor, 2003; Sullivan, 2020):

- **Morning awakening:** Begin your day by gently stimulating your body and mind with herbal alternatives. Trade your coffee for a revitalizing herbal tea like ginseng or peppermint; this means no more morning jitters from too much caffeine! Ginseng offers a natural boost to your central nervous system, promoting mental focus and energy without the crash associated with caffeine. Peppermint tea greets you with a refreshing zing, stimulates digestion, and helps clear morning fog.
- **Culinary creations:** Make your meals an opportunity to introduce herbs that not only enrich flavor but also offer health benefits. Mix fresh cilantro into your guacamole for a detoxifying twist, or blend sage into your butter for an aromatic spread that boosts both memory and taste.
- **Mindful self-care:** Rejuvenate your skincare practice with herbal products. Expand beyond aloe vera to include rose petals for moisture, healing calendula, and toning witch hazel. Design skincare treatments suited to your needs, like a green tea mist for antioxidant protection or a neem leaf soak for its purifying

qualities, or you can start with something simple like adding a few drops of lavender oil to your moisturizer.

- **Clean and green:** Transform your cleaning routine by making your herbal solutions. Try rosemary-infused vinegar for a cleanser that clears the mind with its aroma. Combine one part rosemary-infused vinegar with two parts water for an effective and all-natural surface cleaner. Discover the antifungal benefits of thyme by using it in a lemon-thyme mixture to clean windows and brighten your living space with its uplifting scent.

- **Evening wind-down:** As the evening approaches, encourage relaxation with herbs known for their calming effects. Introduce a pre-sleep ritual with teas like skullcap and lemon balm to ease into restfulness. For some aromatic comfort, add hop flowers to a small pillow or sleep sachet to promote a peaceful night's sleep.

When we include these herbal routines in our lives, we create an environment that benefits our health and happiness. How will you choose to work herbs into your day-to-day routine?

Herbs for Everyday

How else can we invite more of nature into our day? Here, we discover some unique, underrated herbs that can improve sleep quality, support digestive health, and help us manage stress better (*American Herbal Pharmacopoeia*, 2023; Sullivan, 2020).

For Peaceful Slumbers

When the night comes, and sleep doesn't come easily, nature's own selection of herbs can be a gentle solution. Here are two botanicals other than lavender and chamomile that can help you achieve a peaceful night's sleep, enhancing your bedtime routine with their calming properties:

- **Passionflower (*Passiflora incarnata*):** This plant is not only visually striking but also holds compounds that could assist in combating insomnia. Prepare tea from the dried leaves and flowers for a calming pre-sleep drink. Enjoy it about an hour before bed, letting its gentle floral essence set the stage for relaxation.
- **Hops (*Humulus lupulus*):** Beyond their use in the beer industry, hops have qualities that can contribute to a good night's sleep. Although their bitter taste may not be suitable for tea, placing a small pouch of dried hops near your pillow can be soothing, as their fragrance is thought to promote sleep.

For Digestive Harmony

We can't deny that a well-functioning digestive system is funda-mental to our overall well-being, and the botanical world offers critical ingredients for its care. Below are more herbs that can gently restore digestive balance, offering natural and palatable solutions.

- **Lemon balm (*Melissa officinalis*):** This herb, with its inviting citrus fragrance, can help soothe digestive discomfort. For a cold infusion, steep the leaves in cool water for a few hours and drink throughout the day. It is incredibly refreshing when your digestion needs a gentle boost.

- **Dandelion root (*Taraxacum officinale*):** Often dismissed as a simple lawn weed, dandelion root is excellent for digestion. A tea made from roasted dandelion root serves as a mild liver tonic, aiding in digestion and providing a rich, coffee-like taste without caffeine.

Add a teaspoon of honey if you like your beverages on the sweeter side.

For Stress Relief

Ah, yes. Stress is an inevitable part of modern life, but nature provides a way to mitigate its effects. We highlight some uncommon herbs that offer a calming influence on our minds and strengthen the body's resilience:

- **Holy basil (*Ocimum sanctum*):** Known in Ayurvedic practice as Tulsi, this herb is celebrated for its adaptogenic qualities, which help the body to better adapt to stress. Keep a small jar of holy basil on your desk; simply open it and take a deep breath. It can be a quick stress reliever during a hectic day! A warm cup of holy basil tea can be deeply soothing, as its aromatic profile helps to rebalance stress levels.
- **Ashwagandha (*Withania somnifera*):** The roots of ashwagandha, with their distinctive earthy taste, are ideal in a warm, milky mixture before bed or as a morning supplement in its powder form. It is traditionally revered for strengthening the nervous system and stress resilience.

The skill of using herbs effectively is to combine them thoughtfully into your daily habits. Let this guide encourage you to broaden your knowledge and use herbal remedies for a well-balanced approach to natural health.

Mindfulness in Herbal Practice: Cultivating Intuition

In the nurturing space of herbalism, mindfulness is akin to the light that fosters our bond with plant partners, enhancing both their effectiveness and our understanding of them. Developing intuition in this field is about nurturing a unique relationship with herbs that expands beyond their recognized applications. It involves paying attention to the little things—noticing how your body reacts to different herbs and the insights that emerge in moments of quiet and focus. Introducing specific herbal recipes designed to enhance intuition can amplify this mindfulness practice. For instance, preparing a blend of dried blue lotus flower, lavender, and chamomile for tea or a bath can be a deeply meditative process, allowing for a serene state in which one's intuition may flourish (Cassie, 2020; *Matthew Wood Institute of Herbalism*, 2023; Pande, 2021).

Herbal Meditation Practices

Within the quiet of meditation, herbs such as calming blue lotus, lavender, and chamomile become more than supplements; they connect us to heightened awareness. The methodical preparation of these herbs into tea becomes a ritual, fostering a space where mindfulness and intuition intersect. As one ingests the tea or immerses oneself in a bath infused with these ingredients, there is an opening for the calmness required for intuitive work (Cassie, 2020). This practice of intuitive herbalism is about being entirely present with the effect the herb has on your internal experience.

Journaling Your Herbal Experiences

Accompany your sensory explorations with a journal, turning herbal practices into a journey of self-discovery. When journaling, one might reflect on the calming influence of an intuition tea or the protective aura of a mugwort and lavender smoke blend. These experiences, along with the immediate physical reactions and deeper emotional responses, build a comprehensive guide to your herbal intuition journey. Don't know where to start with journaling? Begin by listing the herbs you've used each day and any changes in mood or energy you felt.

Guided Meditation Scripts

To further enhance our intuitive connection with herbs, guided meditation scripts can focus on the qualities of specific plants, like the protective nature of cedarwood or the clarity provided by rosemary and peppermint, both of which have been associated with the third eye chakra and intuitive work (Cassie, 2020; Weed, 2023). Through these meditations, we can explore the plants' symbolic and literal influences on their mindfulness practice.

Interactive Exercises to Engage the Senses

Interactive exercises, such as creating personalized sprays for intuition with essential oils of rosemary, peppermint, and cedarwood, allow for a multi-sensory engagement that can enhance your intuitive abilities, so be sure to spritz some whenever you need a boost of clarity. These sprays can clear the mind and inspire before undertaking intuitive practices (Cassie, 2020). Such hands-on activities not only create a product for further mindfulness but also deepen the intuitive dialogue between practitioner and herb (Hoshaw, 2021).

Aligning With Natural Rhythms

Harmonizing with natural rhythms is enriched by the use of herbs that correspond to these cycles. For instance, the new moon's sense of beginning can be enhanced by the energizing essence of rosemary, while the full moon's culmination might resonate better with the tranquility of chamomile. Using specific herbs in sync with lunar and seasonal changes encourages a reconnection with ancient wisdom and the cycles of the natural world, thereby encouraging an environment where your intuition can grow (Cassie, 2020; Pande, 2021).

Each sip of intuition tea, each breath in a meditative space scented by an intuition smoke blend, and each spritz of an intuitive spray becomes an opportunity to deepen our mindful connection with our inner self and the natural world.

Your Herbal Wellness Plan

You might be feeling unsure of where to start, so here's a roadmap. Begin by selecting the foundational herbs that support your daily wellness. Opt for peppermint to refresh your mornings and sharpen your focus, and consider nettles to enrich your body with vital nutrients. Then, add adaptogens to your routine to cultivate balance and strength. Schisandra berry, in particular, offers dual benefits, boosting your stress resilience and supporting liver function. Gotu kola is excellent when you need cognitive support, especially during the mental exertion needed to complete that project before the deadline or to study for an upcoming exam!

As the day winds down, embrace rituals that promote restoration. Enjoy oat straw tea, a mild nerve tonic, to transition into calmness. On nights when sleep seems just out of reach, a small dose of *Rhodiola rosea* tincture can aid in establishing healthy sleep cycles, ensuring you wake up refreshed and ready for the day ahead.

Think of your wellness approach as a dynamic guide that grows and adjusts with you. Consistently evaluate and adjust your herbal choices to align with your needs (*David Winston's Center for Herbal Studies*, 2023). Be sure to keep a record of how each herb affects you, fine-tuning your daily practices to create a wellness routine that is personal to you.

Living in Harmony With Herbs

As we reach the end of this chapter, I hope that you feel inspired to integrate the herbal knowledge you've gained into your lifestyle with more peace of mind. Consider the subtle strengths of lesser-known herbs, such as the stress-relieving lemon balm or the resilient ashwagandha, which can support you through life's changes, such as the curveballs and unexpected events we can't possibly plan for.

Allow these insights to help you thrive on a personal journey of becoming one with nature. Welcome the embrace of the herbal world, and let your life be enhanced by the sheer delight of connecting with your botanicals.

Chapter 7

The Broader World of Herbalism
Future and Community

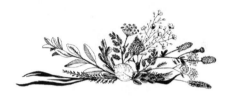

Herbs are the gentle healers of the world.

— Barbara Griggs

H erbs have long been recognized as "gentle healers of the world," and this chapter zeroes in on the expanding influence of herbalism from intimate community roots to its place in the global setting. We glimpse how herbal practices encourage community well-being, evolve through education, and prosper through sustainable and technological innovation.

The chapter discusses the growing recognition of herbal medicine in society and the pivotal role of education in shaping knowledgeable practitioners. It underscores the importance of sustainable and ethical practices in the industry and highlights the interconnectedness of herbalists worldwide in preserving and evolving the craft.

Technological advancements are acknowledged for propelling herbalism into the future alongside the essential community spirit that bolsters the field through symposiums, mentorship, and advocacy.

In essence, this chapter imagines a future in which herbalism combines established practices with cutting-edge research to preserve its modern relevance and therapeutic effectiveness. Now, let's find your fellow herbalists!

Strengthening Connections Through Community

At the heart of every community is the intrinsic power of connection and restoration found in herbalism. This section looks into how the tradition of herbal use surpasses mere health benefits, becoming a crucial aspect of cultural identity within community gardens. We explore how herbalism is intertwined with individual health and the collective vitality of communities worldwide (Vasilis, 2023). Remember when you stumbled on your local herbal workshop and walked away with a new favorite remedy for easing your nerves? It's these small discoveries that enhance our daily wellness practices!

So, how can we then strengthen our connections through community?

Local beginnings and community building:

- Beginnings are often marked by casual gatherings or workshops where herbal secrets and remedies are shared, validating long-standing traditions and knowledge. This might just be where you find the recipe for your new favorite tincture! Practical wisdom passed from neighbor to neighbor.

- These small, intimate settings provide the foundation for larger endeavors, nurturing a space where personal stories and expertise flourish and grow.

The global expansion of herbalism through digital platforms:

- Platforms like Instagram and Facebook have become vibrant corners on the internet for herbalism enthusiasts to exchange guidance, narratives, and safeguards.
- Online communities are vital in enhancing the dialogue of understanding and in establishing strong, supportive networks that span across the globe.
- E-commerce has empowered local herbal practitioners to market their handcrafted products globally, providing them with the economic sustainability of their crafts.

Professional networks and global integration:

- Organizations such as the National Association for Holistic Aromatherapy (NAHA) and American Herbalists Guild (AHG) create opportunities for professional collaboration, keeping their members informed of industry trends and promoting events that blend traditional and modern practices where plant lovers unite and discuss the latest leafy trends!
- These organizations show us the intersection of diverse practices can empower a meaningful global herbal community.

The Evolution and Recognition of Herbal Medicine

Looking back through history, the ancient wisdom surrounding herbs remains influential. There is an increased collective respect and recognition for the role of herbal medicine in managing everyday health. The emerging trend toward more holistic and accessible health practices, mainly the Community Supported Herbal Medicine Movement, represents a societal acceptance of natural remedies as integral to daily wellness (*Stafford Madeer,* 2023).

Educational Pathways in Herbalism

We know that education is essential for developing our expertise, and the same goes for growing our confidence in herbalism. Just as you're now learning what herbalism is, you're expanding your understanding, ensuring the safe and efficient use of herbs; there are renowned organizations like Mountain Rose Herbs that offer comprehensive courses that prepare us to practice herbalism more proficiently. Additionally, ambitions like the Herbalista mobile clinics help share herbal knowledge, enhancing accessibility and community health.

There is a broader range of educational opportunities available for those fascinated by herbalism and who want to uncover more than the foundations:

- **Accredited institutions,** such as the Maryland University of Integrative Health, offer formal programs that blend scientific and traditional knowledge, developing your proficiency in botany, phytochemistry, and clinical application.
- **Professional bodies** like the American Herbalists Guild also advance our professional excellence by

offering certifications that necessitate ongoing
education, adherence to the latest research, and other
sustainable practices.

Sustainability and Ethical Considerations

Sustainable practices are at the core of responsible herbalism. Gaia Herbs demonstrates this commitment through its dedication to environmental stewardship and ensuring its operations contribute positively to our planet and, so, our personal health. This principle underpins the broader societal role of herbalism, reinforcing the idea that each botanical product should be created with respect for the Mother Nature that provides it (*Gaia Herbs*, 2021).

Connecting With Professional Herbalists and Resources

Connecting with experienced herbalists is crucial for deepening one's understanding of plant-based healing. The American Herbalists Guild, for instance, offers a directory to locate credible herbalists and endorses reliable online retailers, thus guaranteeing that the quality of herbs procured is a matter of informed choice (Hoshaw, 2021).

Lifelong Learning: Advanced Studies and Specialization

There is so much more to this art! The field of herbalism encourages endless learning and possibilities for specialization. Initial education might begin with basic courses, like an Herb 101 class, from local schools or online platforms such as The Herbal Medicine Academy that allow for flexible learning. However, your educational journey could continually advance into more specialized fields like clinical herbalism or ethnobotany, encompassing extensive coursework, clinical experience, and research masterclasses.

Herbalism in the Public Sphere

The synergy of herbalism with conservation initiatives is signified by entities like United Plant Savers, whose mission exceeds preserving native medicinal plants to ingraining the understanding and use of these plants within our societal perspectives. They advocate for and implement sustainable harvesting methods that are crucial to maintaining the biodiversity that serves as the foundation of our herbalism practices (*United Plant Savers*, 2022).

Their advocacy reaches into policy and education, emphasizing the importance of plant-based remedies to legislators and arguing for the right to practice herbalism without excessive restrictions. This advocacy takes on heightened significance in a world where striking a balance between human needs and the integrity of nature is increasingly fragile.

Organizations like United Plant Savers are much needed in local education, delivering workshops and producing materials stimulating our eco-conscious engagement with plant life. We need to take better care of our planet and the life that inhabits it, and this includes plants!

Practical Engagement With Herbalism

How do we apply all of this knowledge to building or sustaining a thriving community practically? Active involvement and connectivity with the herbalism community can be achieved through various hands-on experiences:

- **Participate in workshops and plant identification walks:** Does your neighborhood or city have regular plant days? Consider joining local events that provide invaluable knowledge from experienced herbalists. It

An Introduction to Herbalism

can be an excellent venue for experiential learning, community networking, and a way to make eco-minded friends!

- **Attend herbalism conferences:** These gatherings usually offer a wealth of current research and methodologies, keeping practitioners, such as ourselves, up-to-date on advancements within the herbalism discipline.
- **Engage with community gardens:** Ready to get your hands dirty? Direct experience growing and gathering herbs guided by educational programs on herb recognition and crafting herbal preparations is priceless.

Here is how you can go the extra mile to incorporate herbs into your daily routine besides by practicing the art:

- **Harness educational materials:** A vast collection of books and digital content that caters to diverse interests within herbalism, assisting in the awareness and implementation of its principles.
- **Connect with online herbalism groups:** Digital forums and social media groups centered on herbalism provide a wealthy source of guidance, shared experiences, and communal support. Don't be afraid to ask them how they made that enchanting herbal-infused tea.
- **Take part in interactive herb databases:** These tools are invaluable for researching various herbs and their applications and are beneficial for educational and practical exercises. Perfect for settling those "What's this plant?" debates.

By actively participating in these initiatives and harnessing the available tools, we can meaningfully weave herbalism into our lifestyle, improving our personal health, supporting sustainable practices, and developing a stronger connection to the natural world. Who knew going green could be so much fun?

Planting Seeds for the Future

What about future generations? Educational programs oriented toward younger people are essential to maintain the cultural relevance of our herbal practices.

These initiatives might include:

- **Herbal education in schools:** Integrating herbal studies into existing curricula to give students a foundation in botanical knowledge.
- **Interactive youth programs:** Implementing programs in botanical gardens and nature reserves that engage children and teens with the natural world.

The Herb Society of America is among the organizations that provide scholarships and materials to encourage youth interest in herbalism and offer summer programs, internships, and workshops to nurture an appreciation for plant traditions and the environment.

Below are other ways we can cultivate a brighter future for herbalism:

Sustainable Practices for Herbal Stewardship

- **Ethical cultivation:** Embracing practices that ensure the long-term viability of herbal plants, particularly endangered ones. Be sure to read which herbs are on the list (United Plant Savers, 2022). Here are a few on the "at-risk" and "to-watch" lists: American Ginseng (*Panax quinquefolius*), Black Cohosh (*Actaea racemosa*), Echinacea (*Echinacea spp.*), Eyebright (*Euphrasia spp.*), Goldenseal (*Hydrastis canadensis*), Slippery Elm (*Ulmus rubra*).

- **Industry responsibility:** Prioritizing habitat conservation, organic farming, and fair trade to meet increasing herbal product demands responsibly (*American Herbal Products Association*, 2022).
- **Eco-friendly packaging:** Using renewable resources in product packaging and distribution to reduce environmental impact. Hello, paper plates, bamboo cups, and glass jars!

Collaborative Efforts

- **Interdisciplinary strategies:** Working with conservationists and agricultural experts to create a sustainable balance between business interests and ecological health.
- **Conservation initiatives:** Establishing herb sanctuaries, seed banks, and breeding programs to secure the survival of at-risk plant species.

As an herbalist enthusiast, you can support ecological health by partnering with local conservationists and gardeners to promote sustainable herb cultivation and help establish community seed libraries or gardens that preserve "at-risk" plants.

The Green Glow

Advancing Herbalism With Technology

- **Digital tools:** Try apps like PictureThis or iNaturalist for plant identification, and look for lab analysis features within them to judge herbal quality.
- **Scientific research:** Keep updated with the latest studies on herbal efficacy by checking databases such as PubMed or following the Journal of Herbal Medicine.
- **Supply chain integrity:** Blockchain for supply chain ensures that each step from plant harvesting to your shelf is recorded and can be traced back for authenticity; companies like Provenance and VeChain are examples of platforms offering this technology.

Community and Synergy as Central Pillars

The herbalism community thrives on its unity and shared knowledge!

- **Symposiums and celebrations:** Partake in events like the International Herb Symposium or local herb festivals that celebrate plant medicine and bring enthusiasts together.
- **Mentorship programs:** Look for apprenticeships or mentorship opportunities with established herbalists through organizations like the American Herbalists Guild or regional herbalism schools.
- **Public health integration:** Get involved by advocating for the inclusion of herbal options at local health clinics or wellness centers and participating in public forums to discuss the benefits of integrating herbal medicine.

The future of herbalism hinges on both preserving ancient wisdom through education and embracing sustainable and technological advances, ensuring this practice remains relevant and beneficial for generations to come.

Cultivating an Herbal Legacy

As we come to the end of our exploration through herbalism, it becomes evident that the healing potential of plants has not withered over time. The number of herbalists, enthusiasts, and supporters is increasing as more people come to understand the immense value of herbal knowledge.

Herbalism has an extensive history as a therapeutic art, and its continued success depends on the care and attention given to this community, respect for tradition, and openness to new ideas. You can help make the world a better place by doing what you can at home, in your community, and through advocacy for transformation.

Together, we have the opportunity and responsibility to manage this garden of knowledge and create a lasting legacy that will serve as a source of energy and motivation for our future generations.

Conclusion

Your Herbal Journey Ahead

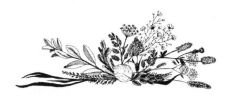

In a way, magic is the act of making a wish come about. Like praying, like plotting, like herbs, like exerting your will on the world, making something happen.

— Philippa Gregory

In the quiet moments following the end of *An Introduction to Herbalism*, it becomes clear that the final sentence is not a period but a comma, signaling a brief pause before leading to an open door of further exploration. This guide, with its comprehensive chapters, has laid out the fundamentals of herbalism, threading together time-honored herbal wisdom with the growing need for holistic health practices in our modern world.

From unraveling the complexities of plant chemistry to offering sage advice on how you can cultivate your own garden and effectively create your own herb remedies, this guide has inspired the variety of ways nature can become part of our daily lives and help restore a sense of balance that is so easily lost during the rush of "getting things done."

Now, with this foundational knowledge, the invitation goes beyond this last page. You are not just a reader anymore but a practitioner encouraged to step into the living practice of herbalism. This book serves as your beginning to a green way of living, nudging you to craft your own course through the expanding fields of herbal remedies. How will your herbal story unfold? Will you seek out a like-minded community in your midst or advocate for a more natural way of living online?

This ongoing process of discovery and sharing has the potential to spark a collective awakening and encourage more and more individuals to reconnect with the natural world, and the wellness it offers is endless!

As you create your own innovations, be it a unique tea blend, a soothing balm, or a tincture, by sharing your insights, you contribute to a collective understanding, maintaining a community that values health, sustainability, and respect for the living world. The story of herbalism is ever-unfolding, and you are now a part of it.

Standing at this entryway, consider the paths before you. Take a moment to reflect on your journey through these pages. How has your perspective shifted? What practices resonate most with you? How will you do more of that? Your personal reflections will guide your steps as you grow into your role as an herbalist.

To further your learning and engagement with herbalism and to join a community where every voice matters, consider this your exclusive invitation to our vibrant Facebook group, "Herbs, Hearts, and Healing." This group is a gathering space for those who share a passion for nature's wisdom and a commitment to wellness. Our rapidly growing community is a cornerstone of our brand, offering you the unique opportunity to connect with fellow herbal enthusiasts, exchange your ideas, and receive a boost of motivation on your journey. By joining, you become part of an inspiring community dedicated to exploring the endless opportunities that herbal remedies bring. A world of support and shared knowledge is just a click away! Witness your herbal practice thrive among friends.

Thank you for embracing The Green Glow as your ally on this enlightening expedition into herbalism. May you continue to nurture this bond with the healing herbs of the Earth and find your healthiest, most vibrant self. As our guide concludes, consider leaving a review to share how this journey has impacted you. What lessons will you carry with you as you continue your practice? Your feedback is valuable as it not only helps us improve and refine but also allows others to find their own path in the natural healing embrace of herbalism.

A final thought: Continuously seek out new information, be open to change, and adapt as science and traditions evolve. May your path be magical and evergreen!

Thanks For Reading!

Hey! Thanks for taking the time to read this and may the seeds of knowledge we've planted grow and flourish. One last thing, and at this point we probably sound like a broken record, but it would mean a great deal to us if you left a review. Also, don't forget to grab your freebie if you haven't already! Just scan the code below. See you in the Facebook group!

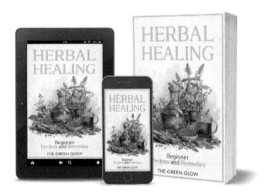

Yes, I almost forgot my freebie

Bibliography

Adaes, S. (2018, August 12). *Rhodiola rosea: medicinal use & science behind it.* Organic Boost. https://organicboost.com/rhodiola-rosea-medicinal-use/

American Botanical Council. (2023). *The ABC clinical guide.* Herbal gram. https://www.herbalgram.org/resources/abc-clinical-guide/

American Herbal Pharmacopoeia. (2023). American Herbal Pharmacopoeia. https://herbal-ahp.org/

American Herbal Products Association. (2022). Ahpa.org. https://www.ahpa.org/

American Herbalists Guild. (2013, June 2). *Herbal medicine faqs.* https://www.americanherbalistsguild.com/herbal-medicine-fundamentals

Badger, A. (2018, November 8). *3 ways to tap into an herbal community near you.* Urban Moonshine. https://www.urbanmoonshine.com/blogs/blog/3-ways-to-tap-into-an-herbal-community-near-you

Better Health Channel. (2021). *Herbal medicine.* https://www.betterhealth.vic.gov.au/health/conditionsandtreatments/herbal-medicine

Brinkley, E. (2022, October 10). *Optimizing social connection with herbs.* Dancing Willow Herbs. https://dancingwillowherbs.com/blogs/news/optimizing-social-connection-with-herbs

Canivenc-Lavier, M.-C. & Bennetau-Pelissero, C. (2023). Phytoestrogens and health effects. *Nutrients, 15*(2), 317-317. https://doi.org/10.3390/nu15020317

Cassie. (2020, March 11). *3 herbal recipes to enhance your intuition:* Zennedout. https://zennedout.com/3-herbal-recipes-to-enhance-your-intuition/

Champagne, É., Royo, A. A., Tremblay, J. & Raymond, P. (2019). Phytochemicals involved in plant resistance to leporids and cervids: a systematic review. *Journal of Chemical Ecology, 46*(1), 84–98. https://doi.org/10.1007/s10886-019-01130-z

Charlemagne. (n.d.). *Charlemagne quotes.* Quote Fancy. https://quotefancy.com/quote/1710220/Charlemagne-Herbs-are-the-friend-of-the-physician-and-the-pride-of-cooks

Chappell, S. (2019, February 21). *A beginner's guide to making herbal salves and lotions.* Healthline Media. https://www.healthline.com/health/diy-herbal-salves

Bibliography

Charles Sturt University. (2023). *Virtual herbarium*. Science Health CSU. https://science-health.csu.edu.au/herbarium

Corinne, J. (2021, June). *5 must have wellness teas to have in your pantry*. SKN Clinic. https://sknclinic.ca/2021/06/01/5-must-have-wellness-teas-to-have-in-your-pantry/

David Winston's Center for Herbal Studies. (2023). Herbal studies. https://herbalstudies.net/

DeJohn, S. (2023). *Herbs for health*. Garden. https://garden.org/learn/articles/view/2236/Herbs-for-Health/

Emerson, R. W. (n.d.). *Ralph Waldo Emerson quotes*. Fsm statistics. https://fsmstatistics.fm/plants-quotes/

Fletcher, J. (2019, January 10). *What is an herbal tincture? Recipes and uses*. Medical News Today. https://www.medicalnewstoday.com/articles/324149

World class botanical events and education for free! (2013). Free herbalism project. https://freeherbalismproject.com/

Gaia Herbs. (2021). Gaia Herbs. https://www.gaiaherbs.com/

Gladstar, R. (n.d.). *Rosemary Gladstar quotes*. Good reads. https://www.goodreads.com/search?utf8=%E2%9C%93&q=Rosemary+Gladstar&search_type=quotes

Gopal, S., Ajgaonkar, A., Kanchi, P., Kaundinya, A., Thakare, V., Chauhan, S., & Langade, D. (2021). Effect of an ashwagandha (Withania Somnifera) root extract on climacteric symptoms in women during perimenopause: A randomized, double-blind, placebo-controlled study. *Journal of Obstetrics and Gynaecology Research*, 47(12), 4414-4425.

Gregory, P. (n.d.). *Philippa Gregory quotes*. Good reads. https://www.goodreads.com/quotes/491242-in-a-way-magic-is-the-act-of-making-a

Griggs, B. (n.d.). *Barbara Griggs quotes*. Fsm statistics. https://fsmstatistics.fm/herbalist-quotes/

Güçlü-Üstündağ, Ö., & Mazza, G. (2023). *Saponins: properties, applications and processing*. Critical Reviews in Food Science and Nutrition. https://www.tandfonline.com/doi/abs/10.1080/10408390600698197

Healthline. (2017, October 30). *Homegrown herbal remedies*. Healthline Media. https://www.healthline.com/health/herbal-remedies-from-your-garden

Herbal Encyclopedia. (2010, December 30). *Cross reference scientific names of herbs with common names easily*. https://cloverleaffarmherbs.com/scientific-names/

Hippocrates. (2019, December 18). *Hippocrates quotes*. Wise owl quotes. https://wiseowlquotes.com/hippocrates/

Hoshaw, C. (2021, May 14). *Herbal medicine 101: how you can harness the power of healing herbs*. Healthline Media. https://www.healthline.-com/health/herbal-medicine-101-harness-the-power-of-healing-herbs

Iannotti, M. (2022). *Types of mulch and why you should use them*. The Spruce. https://www.thespruce.com/what-is-mulch-1402413

Jekyll, G. (2023). *Gertrude Jekyll quotes*. Brainy Quote. https://www.brainyquote.com/quotes/gertrude_jekyll_310275

Jones, T. (2017, October 20). *10 healthy herbal teas you should try*. Healthline Media. https://www.healthline.com/nutrition/10-herbal-teas

Kolen, R. (2022). *5 tips for preserving homemade & natural body care products*. Mountain Rose Herbs. https://blog.mountainroseherbs.com/5-tips-preserving-handcrafted-natural-bodycare-products

Littefield, S. (2023). *Nutrition you can grow in your garden*. Garden. https://garden.org/learn/articles/view/3856/Nutrition-You-Can-Grow-In-Your-Garden/

Matthew Wood Institute of Herbalism. (2023). https://www.matthewwoodinstituteofherbalism.com/

Moorhouse, D. (2018, June 30). *Ancient Egyptian medicine*. Schools History. https://schoolshistory.org.uk/topics/medicine-through-time/ancient-egyptian-medicine/

Moss, W. (2023). *Starting plants from seed*. Garden. https://garden.org/learn/articles/view/4433/Starting-Plants-From-Seed/

Mountain rose herbs. (2022). *How herbalism helps communities blossom*. https://blog.mountainroseherbs.com/herbalism-helps-communities

Najafian, Y., Hamedi, S. S., Farshchi, M. K., & Feyzabadi, Z. (2018). Plantago major in traditional Persian medicine and modern phytotherapy: a narrative review. *Electronic Physician*, *10*(2), 6390-6399. https://doi.org/10.19082/6390

National Center for Complementary and Integrative Health. (2023). *Herbs at a glance*. NCCIH. https://www.nccih.nih.gov/health/herbsataglance

National Gardening Association. (2023). Garden. https://garden.org/

Neveln, V. (2016). *15 easy-to-grow herbs that are perfect for beginners*. Better Homes & Gardens. https://www.bhg.com/gardening/vegetable/herbs/easy-to-grow-herbs/

NT Contributor. (2003, August 26). *Herbal remedies: integration into conventional medicine*. Nursing Times. https://www.nursingtimes.net/archive/herbal-remedies-integration-into-conventional-medicine-26-08-2003/

Pan, S.-Y., Litscher, G., Gao, S.-H., Zhou, S.-F., Yu, Z.-L., Chen, H.-Q., Zhang, S.-F., Tang, M.-K., Sun, J.-N., & Ko, K.-M. (2014). Historical perspective of traditional indigenous medical practices: the current renaissance and conservation of herbal resources. *Evidence-Based*

Complementary and Alternative Medicine, 2014(525340), 1-20. https://doi.org/10.1155/2014/525340

Pande, K. (2021, October 29). *Does intuition play a role in modern herbal practice?* Herbal Reality. https://www.herbalreality.com/herbalism/western-herbal-medicine/intuition-herbal-medicine-practice/

Paracelsus. (n.d.). *Paracelsus quotes*. Brainy Quote. https://www.brainyquote.com/quotes/paracelsus_138349

Porta, C. (2023). *Botanical medicines: foundations and practical applications.* Bakken Center for Spirituality & Healing. https://csh.umn.edu/academics/for-credit-courses/csph-5423-botanical-medicines-foundations-and-practical-applications

Richter, C. (2023). *Growing herbs indoors*. Garden. https://garden.org/learn/articles/view/36/Growing-Herbs-Indoors/

Rodale Institute. (2021, January 20). *Free downloadable resources*. https://rodaleinstitute.org/education/resources/

Rosemary Gladstar's science & art of herbalism. (2016, April 13). The Science & Art of Herbalism. https://scienceandartofherbalism.com/

Santos, C. M. M., & Silva, A. M. S. (2020). The antioxidant activity of prenylflavonoids. *Molecules, 25*(3), 696. https://doi.org/10.3390/molecules25030696

Simple Loose Leaf Tea Company. (2020, March 17). *8 simple, homemade herbal tea recipes*. Simple Loose Leaf Tea Company. https://simplelooseleaf.com/blog/herbal-tea/herbal-tea-recipes/

Social impact. (2018). Gaia Herbs. https://www.gaiaherbs.com/pages/social-impact

Sowmya Andole, Thumma, G., Praveen Kumar Kusuma, Narender Boggula, Jainendra Kumar Battineni, Bakshi, V. & Kiran Gangarapu. (2023). Medicinal plants against SARS-CoV/Corona virus infections: ethnopharmacology, chemistry, clinical, and preclinical studies. *Springer EBooks*, 1-24. https://doi.org/10.1007/978-3-030-83350-3_15-1

Stafford Madeer, L. (2023). *The community supported herbal medicine movement*. Herbal gram. https://www.herbalgram.org/resources/herbalgram/issues/88/table-of-contents/hg88orgnews_commherbmed/

Sullivan, J. (2020, August 7). *A delicious summertime mocktail for immunity*. Wish Garden Herbs. https://www.wishgardenherbs.com/blogs/wishgarden/incorporating-herbs-into-your-daily-life

Ruskovska, T., Massaro, M., Maria Annunziata Carluccio, Arola-Arnal, A., Muguerza, B., Wim Vanden Berghe, Declerck, K., Calabriso, N., Combet, E., Gibney, E. R., Gomes, A., Gonthier, M.-È., Kistanova, E., Irèna Krga, Mena, P., Morand, C., Santos, C. N., Sonia de Pascual-Teresa, Rodriguez-Mateos, A., & Egeria Scoditti. (2020). Systematic bioinformatic analysis of nutrigenomic data of flavanols in cell models of cardiometabolic disease. *Food & Function*, *11*(6), 5040-5064. https://doi.org/10.1039/d0fo00701c

TeaUSA. (2013). *Brewing tea.* https://www.teausa.com/14521/brewing-tea

The Botanical Society of America. (2023). CMS Botany. https://cms.botany.org/home.html

The Herb Guide. (2023). *Herbal tea.* https://www.the-herb-guide.com/herbal-tea.html

The history of herbal medicine. (2020). New Chapter. https://www.newchapter.com/wellness-blog/the-history-of-herbal-medicine/

United plant savers. (2022, September 23). https://unitedplantsavers.org/

Vasilis, E. (2023). *The power of herbs in building unity through community gardens: growing together and connecting through nature's bounty.* Coohom. https://www.coohom.com/article/the-power-of-herbs-in-building-unity-through-community-gardens

Wack, M. (2021, August 27). *Types of herbal tea and their benefits.* Artful Tea. https://artfultea.com/blogs/wellness/types-of-herbal-tea-and-their-benefits

Weed, S. (2023). *Herbal medicine: advice, articles, books, workshops, intensives, apprenticeship, correspondence courses.* Susun Weed. http://www.susunweed.com/

World Health Organization. (2019, November 25). *Traditional, complementary and integrative medicine.* https://www.who.int/health-topics/traditional-complementary-and-integrative-medicine#tab=tab_1

Yutang, L. (2023). *Lin Yutang* quotes. Good reads. https://www.goodreads.com/quotes/122552-there-is-something-in-the-nature-of-tea-that-leads

Zhang, L., Virgous, C., & Si, H. (2019). Synergistic anti-inflammatory effects and mechanisms of combined phytochemicals. *Journal of Nutritional Biochemistry*, *69*, 19-30. https://doi.org/10.1016/j.jnutbio.2019.03.009

Made in the USA
Columbia, SC
03 April 2024

33902362R00054